# 101 Muscle-Shaping Workouts & Strategies

FOR WOMEN

# Contents

CHAPTER 7

## 116 GLUTES/LEGS



CHAPTER 8

## 156 SHOULDERS



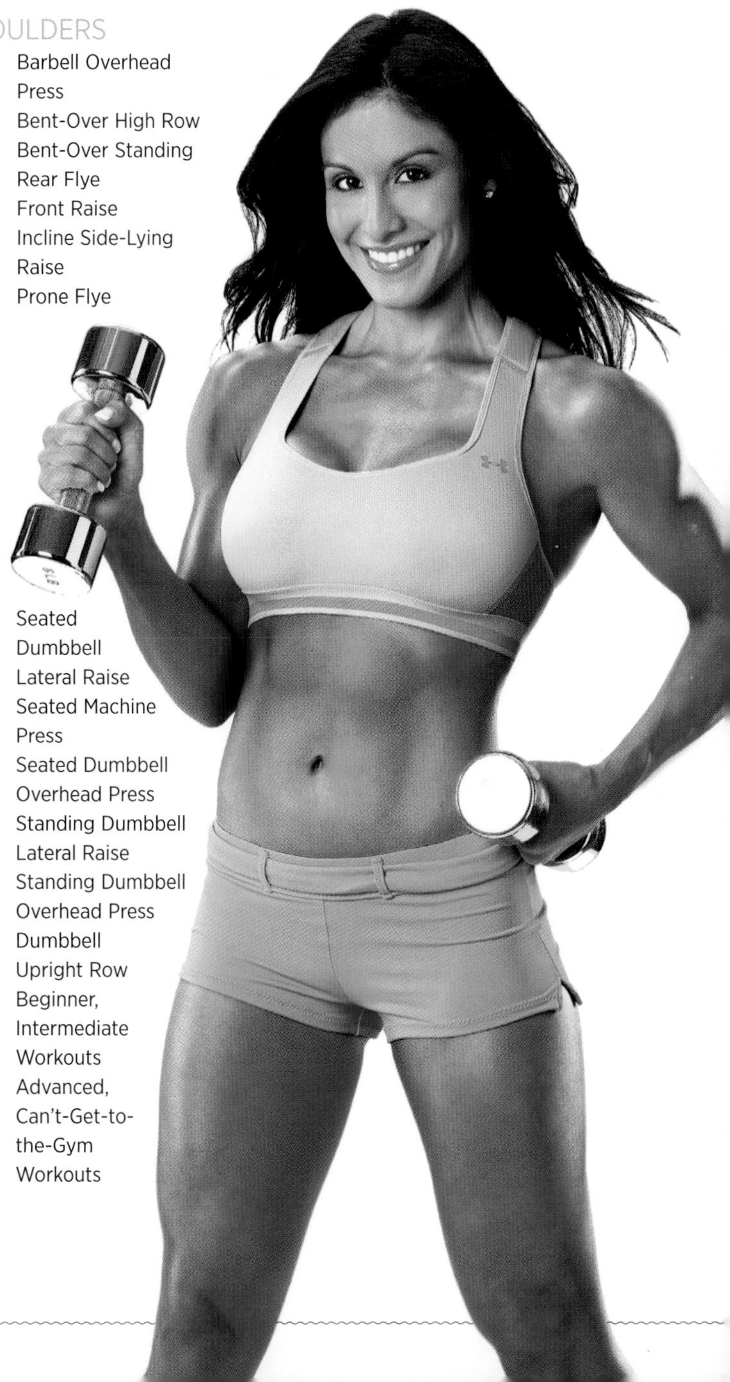

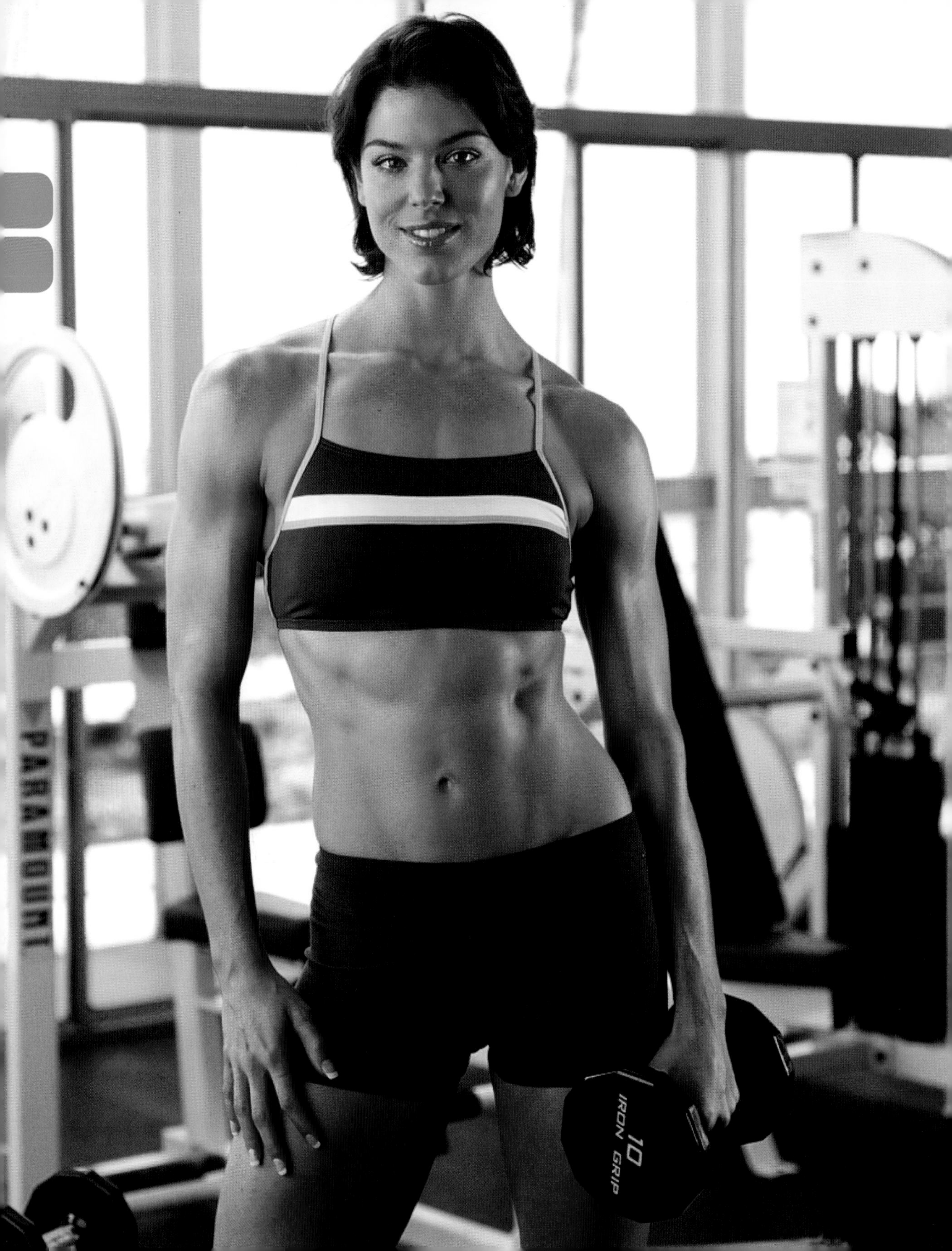
PARAMOUNT
10
IRON GRIP

Chapter 1

# Basic Training

*Whether you're new to the gym or just want to add variety to your program, this is your starting place*

WHAT'S THE FASTEST, most effective way to transform your body? The answer is strength training. Sure, cardiovascular exercise, stretching and good eating habits are important for keeping fit, healthy and trim. But when it comes to sculpting and firming your body, no form of exercise offers more bang for your buck than lifting weights.

Not only can you develop sleek thighs, awesome abs and taut triceps in as little as six weeks, but hitting the weight room regularly can impact your health for years to come. With the right strength-training program, you can bank away precious bone mass, one of the keys to preventing osteoporosis. Having more muscle tissue will also boost your metabolism, increasing your body's capacity to burn calories, even when you're just sitting around. Studies show that strength training can even help combat high blood pressure and cardiovascular disease, as well as perk up your mood, boost your energy level and help you fight stress.

*101 Muscle-Shaping Workouts & Strategies for Women* will help you get the most from your program, whether you're jumping in for the first time or looking for ideas to freshen up an old routine. You'll find all the essential tools, including 100-plus exercises and stretches and specific programming for each bodypart. But that's only part of the package. We'll help you determine which equipment to use, how much weight to lift, how often to work out, how many exercises to perform and how to help you get the body you want. We'll also explain essential training principles and advanced workout techniques to help you progress to the next level. Plus, we'll clear up some misconceptions about lifting weights.

# WHY WEIGHT TRAINING WORKS

If there's one word that explains the remarkable benefits of strength training, it's overload. Change can only happen when you push harder than usual. Overloading your muscles — challenging them with sufficiently heavy weights — stimulates them to grow stronger. The best way to overload is to progressively increase the resistance each time an exercise is no longer challenging, forcing your muscles to respond and develop. You can also progressively overload by manipulating other training variables: the number of sets and reps, exercise selection, order you do them in and the speed at which you perform them. Other related components are exercise frequency, or how many days per week you lift; and recovery, which encompasses how much rest you need between sets, exercises and training sessions. All of these factors are related; your program becomes different just by changing one of them.

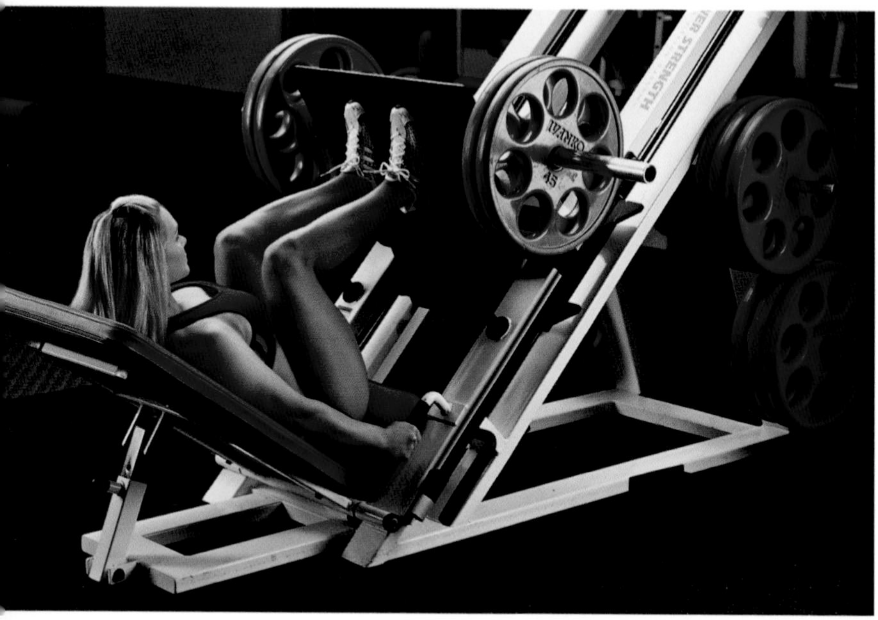


## THE LOWDOWN ON EQUIPMENT

There is no "best" piece of equipment. Dumbbells, barbells, machines and cables: all of these contraptions can help you build strength. You can even get stronger without any equipment at all. Still, in certain circumstances, some equipment is more effective than others, and using a combination will give you the best of all worlds. Here's a rundown of the major equipment options.

### Weight Machines

Don't fret if you look at a machine and can't figure out which way to sit, which handle to pull or which bodypart you're supposed to be exercising. It's not always obvious, which is why most machines feature an illustration and operating instructions. A trainer or experienced lifter can help you adjust the seat and various levers so the machine fits your body. Some machines use weight stacks (therefore called a stack machine), a tall column of weight plates marked in numerical order, as their resistance. Others use loose plates, which are round weights that are usually stored on various weight trees around the gym. Note: all machines are not created equal; different makes that are for the same bodypart vary just as 10 pounds on the chest press might not be the same as 10 pounds on the shoulder press. To avoid injury, test the weight on every machine before using it. Record how much weight you use for each one so you don't have to experiment during your next session. Once you have a starting weight, use this as a base to progress.

**Pros:** Machines don't require much balance or coordination, so a newbie can quickly get the hang of an exercise. You simply get into position and the machine guides you through the motion. (Still, there are subtle technique tips to master.) With no loose parts to drop, machines are extremely safe. They are also ideal for isolating a muscle group — in other words, targeting one muscle group to the exclusion of all others. Machines also allow you to work certain muscle groups from angles that just aren't attainable with other equipment, because your body is stabilized in a particular position and held by the machine so you can safely lift more weight. And to adjust the amount of weight, you simply place a pin in the weight stack.

**Cons:** Although isolating muscle groups can be useful in some cases, it's generally better to work several muscle groups at once, mimicking the way your body operates in everyday life. Because machines keep you in position, they don't demand much of your core muscles, the deep abdominal, lower back and hip muscles that are essential for good posture and are called upon to stabilize your body when you perform other types of exercises. In addition, traditional weight machines are designed for only one or two movements, so they aren't very versatile, although many of the new versions do have pulley systems that allow for multi-plane or multi-directional training.

### Free Weights

A free weight is simply a weight that is not attached to any kind of machine. Free weights — both barbells (the long ones you grip with two hands) and dumbbells (the short ones you grasp with one hand) — come in all shapes and sizes. Free weights require you to use your own muscular strength and good posture to stabilize your body and keep your alignment in check while you perform the exercise. You're responsible for controlling the weight at all times, and your body dictates its path of motion, rate of speed and balance. Although advanced exercisers tend to gravitate toward free weights, with proper guidance there's no reason beginners can't safely use them, too. However, we recommend that novices work with a trainer at least once or twice before tackling free weights solo. Even if you're an experienced lifter, never do any heavy lifting alone. Always enlist a spotter who's ready to grab the bar in case your muscles give out.

**Pros:** Free weights offer a more complete and challenging workout than machines because they work more than just the targeted muscles. For instance, when you do a dumbbell shoulder press, your abdominals and lower back muscles also kick in, keeping your torso stable while your shoulder muscles press up the dumbbells. Plus, free weights allow your joints to move in a way that feels most natural, rather than forcing them to follow the predetermined pathway of a machine. Free weights are versatile, too. With just a few sets of dumbbells, you can perform dozens of

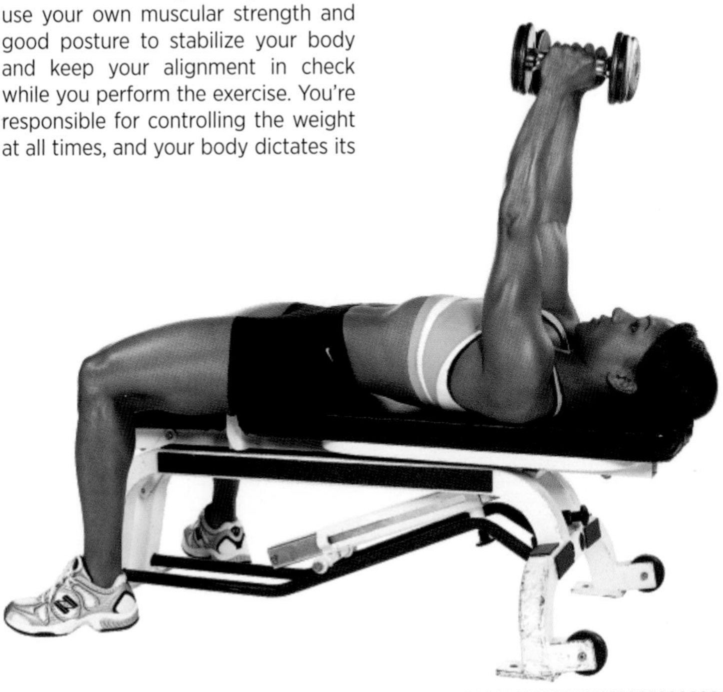

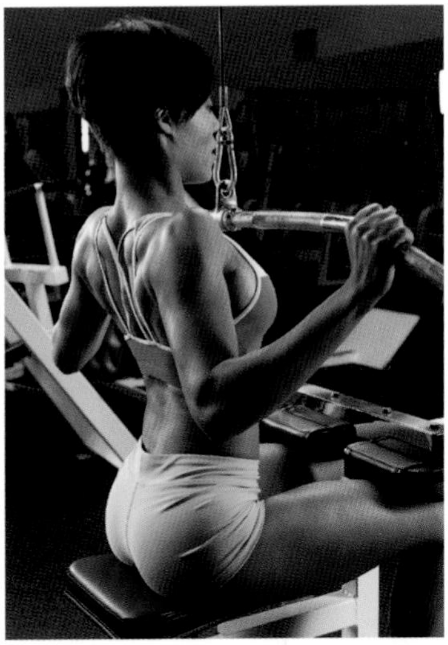

exercises. Add an adjustable weight bench to the mix, and you can expand your repertoire even more.

**Cons:** Free-weight exercises have a higher learning curve than machines and generally require some instruction at first. Also, extra caution should be taken when using free weights, to avoid accidents.

### Cable Machines

Cable machines are sort of a hybrid of machines and free weights. They feature a weight stack, but they are highly versatile. You can perform dozens of exercises on a cable machine by adjusting the height of the pulley so that it's close to the floor, up over your head, or anywhere in between. Also, you can clip a dozen different handles onto the same pulley and instantly create different exercises.

**Pros:** Cable machines aren't as constricting as regular machines. For instance, when you pull a bar to your chest from overhead, as in the lat pulldown, you control the pathway of the bar. This makes the exercises more effective than a similar exercise on a weight machine. You also get resistance in both directions as you lift and lower because you have to resist the pull of the machine on the return. In addition, cable machines provide more safety and stability than free weights, and the exercises are easier to learn.

**Cons:** Unlike weight machines, cables don't have cams, small kidney-shaped pulleys that change the resistance to match what your muscle is able to lift at each point of a movement. (When your muscle has good mechanical advantage, the cam gives it more work to do; when you're at a weak point during the exercise, the cam lightens the load.) Because there's no cam, you may hit points in some exercises where your muscles won't be working to their fullest throughout the motion, as they do with regular machines.

### Additional Strength-Training Tools

Although free weights, machines and cables are the most common types of strength-training equipment, you'll likely come across other devices as well. Some machines are designed so that the resistance comes from air pressure, and you adjust the difficulty of the exercise by punching a number into a computer. Other contraptions look like machines but use free-weight plates instead of a weight stack. A stability ball or medicine ball can also be an excellent strength-training tool. Rubber exercise tubing can provide a significant challenge as well. However, most bodyweight and tubing exercises provide a limited amount of resistance, so as you become stronger, you may need to use machines and free weights.

## THE BUILDING BLOCKS OF A STRENGTH WORKOUT

Strength training is part science, part art. There are certain basic, immutable facts, such as 1) you shouldn't work the same muscle group on consecutive days, and 2) every program should include at least one exercise for every major muscle. However, there's no rule dictating how many days a week you should lift weights, and there's no law stating how many or which specific exercises you need to do. There are simply guiding principles, like the ones in this section, to help you construct a sound workout program that fits your goals, fitness level, schedule and personal preferences.

### REPS AND SETS

A rep — short for repetition — is one full run-through of an exercise, including both the lifting and the lowering phases. The number of reps you perform can have a significant effect on your results. For optimal strength and bone building, experts generally recommend performing 8 to 12 reps. However, you must use enough weight so that your muscles fatigue on the final repetition. If you get to your 12th rep and feel that you could easily crank out a few more, you haven't used enough weight. The last two reps of any set should be very challenging to the point you may have to struggle to complete them with good form. This creates muscle fatigue, which is key to stimulating muscle change. If you tried to do another rep and couldn't even lift the weight without compromising your form, this is

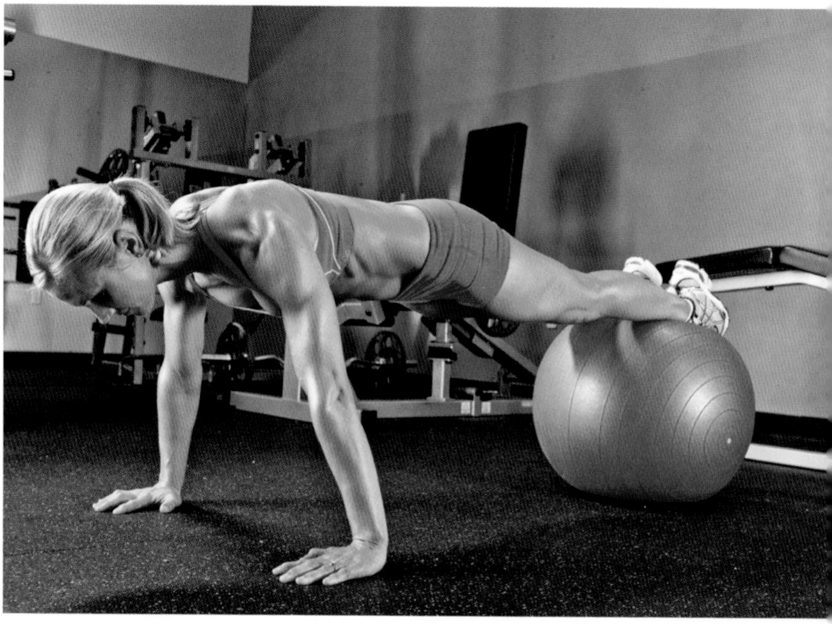

muscle failure; it can also be risky, especially if training alone, so you need to be cautious.

It's a misconception that performing 20–30 reps with light weights will give you tone without bulk. In truth, performing a high number of reps won't provide enough overload to stimulate muscle or bone growth. Performing fewer than eight reps is fine periodically for advanced exercisers who are aiming for maximum strength, but lifting weights that heavy does carry a greater risk of injury, and it's not something that even advanced exercisers should do all the time.

Research suggests the best way to keep progressing is to vary the number of reps you perform. For instance, aim for 10 reps on Monday, 6–8 reps on Wednesday, and 12 reps on Friday, then repeat the cycle. Or, spend three or four weeks aiming for 10 reps, the next month aiming for 6–8 reps, and so on.

For best results, perform each rep slowly, maintaining control of the weight throughout the entire motion. If you zoom through your reps, you'll rely on momentum rather than muscle power and you'll cheat your muscles out of a good workout. A basic rule of thumb: Take two seconds to lift a weight and four seconds to lower it.

A set is a group of consecutive reps typically followed by a brief rest period. It is dependent on the amount of weight you're using. In general, you'll do fewer reps with heavier weight and more reps with lighter weight, although the number of sets may stay the same. One to two sets per muscle group may be sufficient for beginners, but research suggests that after a few months, you're likely to hit a plateau. Eventually, it's a good idea to perform three or four sets per muscle group. However, this doesn't mean you need to do three or four sets of the same exercise. For example, you may want to perform two sets of one chest exercise and two sets of a different one.

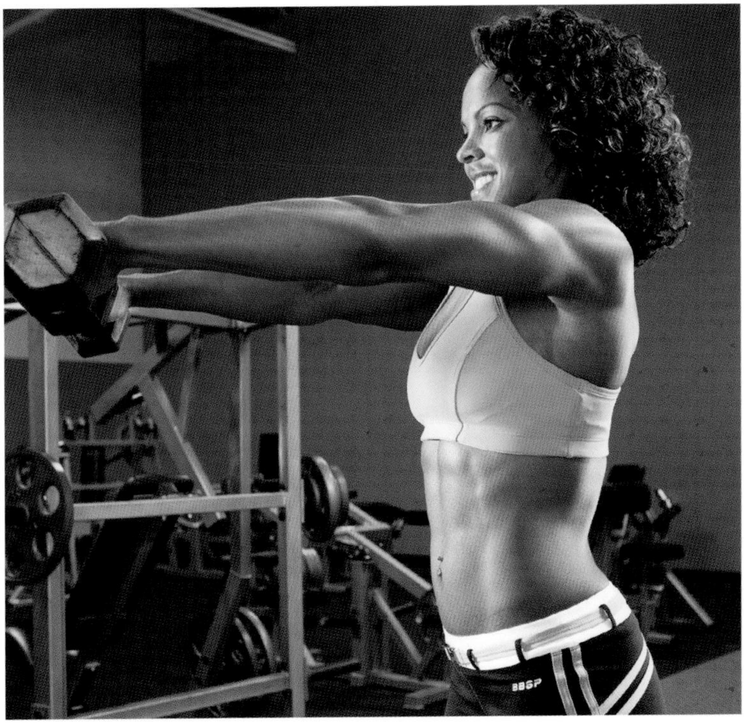

## RESTING BETWEEN SETS

Most people find that 60–90 seconds is enough to feel recovered from a set. As you become more fit, you can gradually decrease your rest periods. However, if you are lifting especially heavy weights, you may need to rest a few minutes before your next set. One of the advanced training techniques described on page 13 — supersets — involves performing two consecutive sets before resting.

## CHOOSING A WEIGHT

You'll choose the amount of weight for each exercise by trial and error. If you're just starting out, choose a weight you believe you can handle, and complete at least eight reps with good form, but not more than 10 reps. If you can accomplish eight reps easily, you need more weight. If you can't complete eight, reduce your weight until you can complete at least eight but no more than 10. You'll need to do this for every exercise and then note when this number of reps gets easy, usually every 3–4 weeks or so, because you'll need to increase your weight when it's no longer challenging. You may find you're increasing weight for some muscle groups and not others, so take note of these different muscular timetables. Also, you may feel stronger on some days than others and should adjust your weights accordingly.

## EXERCISE SELECTION

No matter what your fitness level or time constraints, always strive for balance. In other words, perform at least one exercise for each major muscle group — chest, upper back, middle back, shoulders, biceps, triceps, glutes, quadriceps, hamstrings, abs and lower back. If you overemphasize one group and neglect another, you may increase your risk for injury.

If you're a beginner, don't overwhelm yourself by trying to learn every move. Choose one or two exercises for each muscle group and master them before you tackle others. Be sure to learn the name and purpose of each exercise so that you can design a sensible, balanced workout. Writing this information down in a workout journal will help drill it into your brain.

It's a good idea to start with basic exercises that don't require much balance. For instance, try the chest press machine rather than the dumbbell chest press or barbell bench press. However, don't confine yourself to machines indefinitely; after a few weeks, try out some free weights, too. Include both multijoint (exercises that work more than one muscle at a time, such as squats and lunges), and single-joint exercises, such as leg extensions, in your routine.

As you gain strength and experience, learn new exercises for each muscle group and challenge yourself with multi-muscle moves that require more core strength and coordination. In addition, learn to work each muscle from new angles, and try some of the advanced training techniques described in this chapter.

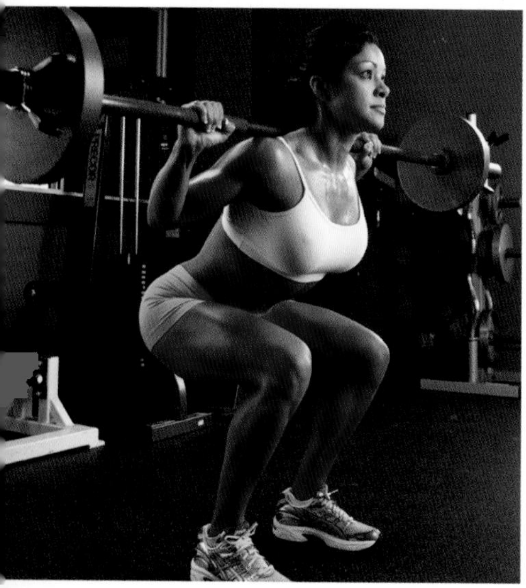

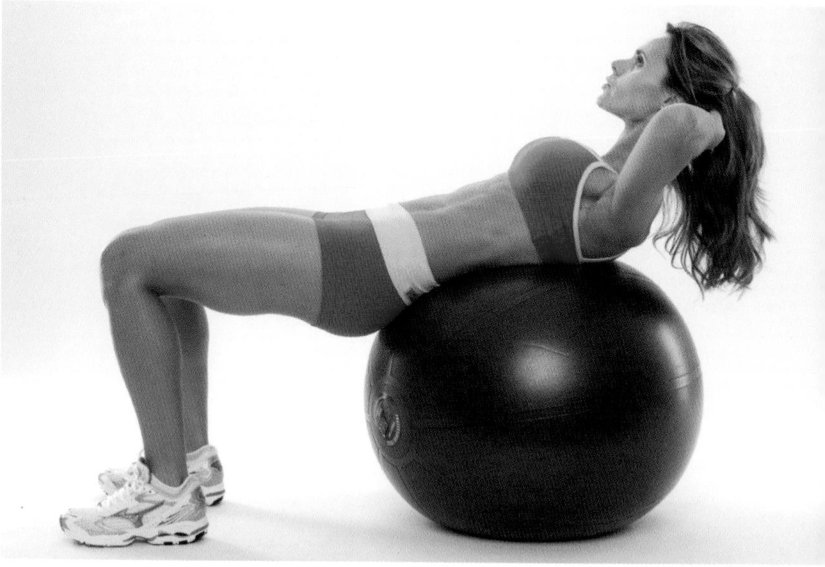

## EXERCISE ORDER

In general, work your larger muscles, such as legs and back, before targeting the smaller muscles that assist them. Typically, this means starting with compound movements, which use more than one muscle group and joint (the chest press, for example), then turning to isolation-type movements, which use only one muscle group and joint (the pec flye). If you do an isolation-type exercise first, chances are that those smaller assisting muscles that you've fatigued will limit your ability to overload the relevant larger muscle groups later. For more advanced routines, if you're doing a high-intensity training workout or splits, start with multi-muscle exercises first, then finish with isolation training. With specific superset and compound set techniques, you may be incorporating both multi-muscle and single-joint isolation exercises as part of one set.

## WORKOUT FREQUENCY

Aim to target each muscle group twice a week on non-consecutive days. Muscles need at least 48 hours to recover from the trauma caused by strength training; without sufficient rest, you'll get weaker instead of stronger. Targeting each muscle group three times a week doesn't offer appreciably better results than lifting twice a week, so you may be better off devoting any extra time to cardiovascular workouts. Also, as you become more advanced and your workouts become more intense, you may need more than one day off between workouts for the same muscle groups.

If you're a beginner, you may want to work all of your muscle groups on the same day. Since you're only doing one or two exercises per muscle group, your workouts may last just 20–30 minutes. However, veterans might want to "split" their routines into four or more days. See the nextpage for more details on split routines.

## INCREASING THE INTENSITY OF YOUR WORKOUTS

The simplest way to increase your intensity is by increasing the load, or the amount of weight you lift. To do this safely, consider your current condition, training background and exercise history when designing a high-intensity program. Because a high-intensity workout is very challenging, beginners should have a good strength base before attempting one. For the best results, your workouts should include heavy and moderate intensities mixed either in a particular session or during the week. You can split a bodypart into heavy and moderate exercises. For chest, for example, do heavy bench presses, moderate dumbbell presses and moderate cable crossovers. Or divide a workout week into a heavy day, rest day, moderate day, active recovery day, heavy day and rest day. Just remember to cycle your bodyparts and exercises so they alternate between the heavy and moderate intensities.

To prevent overuse injuries, the frequency of high-intensity exercise should be limited to no more than once or twice a week per bodypart. Take at least one day of rest between training a particular muscle group, but if muscle soreness persists, you need more rest. You could also schedule an "active recovery" day of light aerobic exercise after a high-intensity total-body resistance workout to enhance recovery. For sufficient muscle stimulation and injury prevention, you need to use moderate weights for 8–12 reps, and a light day once every few weeks can be beneficial, too.

## Getting to the Next Level: ADVANCED TRAINING TECHNIQUES

There's a lot more to getting stronger and firmer than simply lifting heavier weights. It's also important to stimulate more fibers of each muscle. You can do this by attacking each muscle from several angles and by fatiguing your muscles with advanced training techniques. Here are several ways to really blitz your muscles and maximize your results. Think of these options as tools to keep your training workouts and cycles in peak running condition, and make the most of your training time. Variety is not only essential for muscle conditioning, but it also adds to your enjoyment during workouts by keeping things fresh.

### SPLIT ROUTINES

Once you get serious about strength training — adding new exercises and more sets to your program — a total-body routine will start to eat up too much time, and you may start to lose focus by the end of your long workouts. So rather than spend an hour or more in the weight room, divide your routine into two or three shorter workouts. For example, train your upper body twice a week and your lower body on opposite days, adding abs and lower back to either day. Or, try a "push/pull" split routine, separating your upper-body pushing muscles (chest and triceps) from the upper-body muscles involved in pulling motions (back and biceps). Add your lower body and abdominal exercises to either day or do them on a separate day altogether. You'll find several examples of split routines in this book.

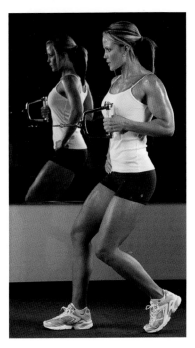

Brief, focused workouts help you stay fresh and motivated. If you walk into the gym knowing that all you have to do that day is work your back, biceps and abs, you're likely to give those muscle groups an all-out effort — the kind of effort that really brings about results.

When designing a split routine, make sure that you hit each muscle group twice a week and you don't work the same muscle group on consecutive days. Also, work your chest and triceps on the same day rather than back-to-back since your triceps get some work during chest exercises. The same goes for your back and biceps.

### SUPERSETS

A superset consists of two different exercises performed consecutively without rest. (A superset consisting of three exercises is sometimes called a tri-set.) A superset can be opposing muscle groups, for example, go immediately from a quadriceps exercise to a hamstring exercise; or, you can superset the same primary muscle, for example doing two quadriceps exercises back-to-back. Another superset combo is compound and isolation movements, for example chest press with an overhead triceps extension. (Both exercises work the triceps, but the second isolates them.) After a rest between supersets, you repeat the superset before moving on to the next one. This pumps up the volume if the same muscle group is worked or it can also aid muscle recovery when opposing muscles are worked because it builds in an active rest for each of the muscle groups. Any superset variation is a great way to speed up your routine.

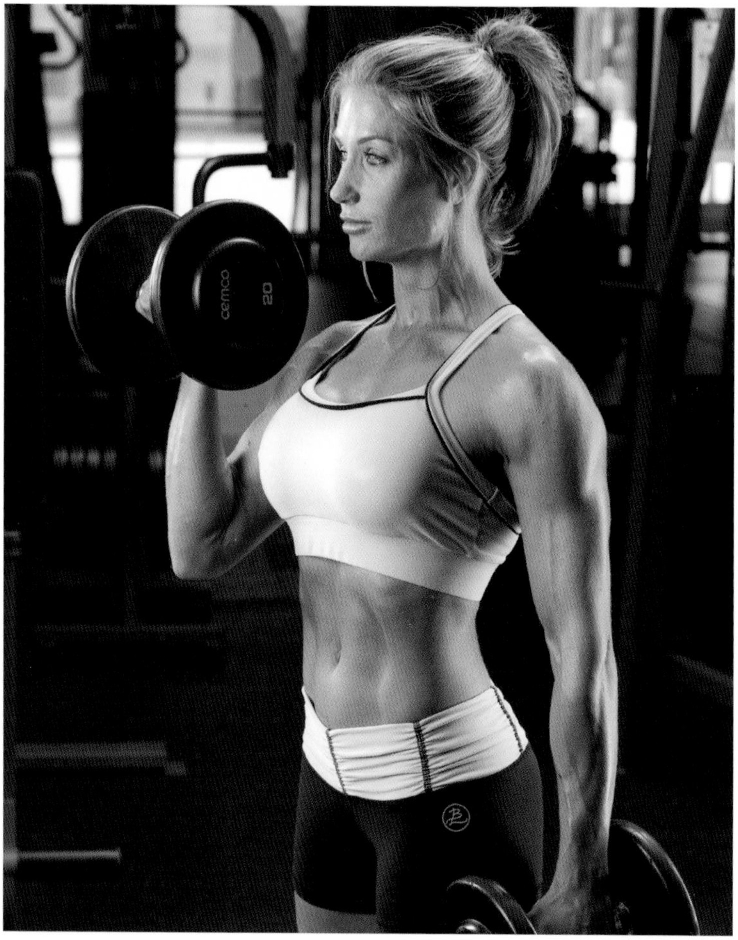


## PYRAMIDS

Do three or more sets of an exercise using progressively heavier weights while performing fewer reps. For instance, start with moderate weight and do a set of 12 reps, then increase the weight and drop to 10 reps, then add more weight and do eight reps. You can reverse the pyramid, moving from high weight and low reps to low weight and high reps, to get the most out of varying your reps and weights.

## DROP SETS

This technique allows you to use heavier weight and then reduce the weight as you become fatigued. Choose a weight that exhausts your muscles after about 10 reps, then immediately drop the weight by 5–20 pounds and try to squeeze out 3–5 more reps to complete the set. It's safer and most efficient to try this technique with machines. By the time you replace the weight plates on a barbell or pick up a new pair of dumbbells, your muscles will already have had some time to recover.

## ➲ ROUTINE: full body

**Frequency:** 2–3 days per week

**Best for:** beginners, intermediates

If you have little experience or are simply in a major time crunch, start with the full-body routine. It's great for general, overall muscle conditioning. Nothing gets overworked, you get plenty of off days for recovery and you work each muscle 2–3 times per week. Full-body training is also very efficient, as your entire body is worked in one session. This way, if you can make it to the gym only once or twice a week, at least every muscle group has been trained. Ideally, aim for 2–3 workouts per week on average.

To design your full-body routine, choose a compound exercise (one that uses multiple joints, like the bench press or leg press) for each muscle group and do 2–4 sets of each exercise. Want to make this routine harder? Try combining two or three exercises at a time into a superset.

### Sample full-body schedule

**Day 1:** full body (chest, shoulders, back, arms, abs, quads, hamstrings/glutes and calves)
**Day 2:** off
**Day 3:** full body
**Day 4:** off
**Day 5:** full body
**Day 6:** off
**Day 7:** off

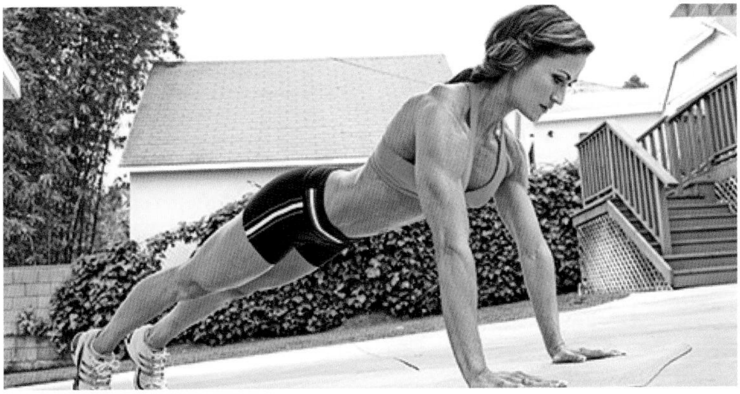

## Sample upper/lower schedule

| 3-day sample | BEGINNER/INTERMEDIATE | 4-day sample | ADVANCE |
|---|---|---|---|
| | Day 1: upper | | Day 1: upper |
| | Day 2: off | | Day 2: lower |
| | Day 3: lower | | Day 3: off |
| | Day 4: off | | Day 4: upper |
| | Day 5: upper | | Day 5: lower |
| | Day 6: off | | Day 6: off |
| | Day 7: off | | Day 7: off |

**Note:** *Start next week with lower*

### ➲ ROUTINE: upper/lower

**Frequency:** 2–4-day split
**Best for:** intermediates

Take your training to the next level by splitting your upper body and lower body into different sessions. As the name implies, you'll do an upper day (chest, shoulders, back, arms) and a lower day (quads, hamstrings/glutes and calves). Choose 1–2 exercises for each major muscle group of the upper body and two exercises for each lower-body muscle group. You can split up your training anywhere from a two-times-weekly routine all the way to a more advanced four-times-weekly routine. The most common method is the every-other-day approach, where you train three times per week and pick back up where you left off the following week. Three days per week is a great way to start. Move to four days per week after following this routine for 4–6 weeks. Include abs at the end of either workout, being sure to train them 2–3 times per week with at least one day in between for rest.

### ➲ ROUTINE: opposing muscle groups

**Frequency:** three-day split
**Best for:** intermediate, advanced

Pair muscle groups together that oppose each other (like chest and back), which puts pulling muscles with pushing muscles in the same workout instead of splitting them up on different days. Major benefit: one muscle gets worked while the opposing one rests. This allows for efficient workouts because you can move quickly from one exercise to the next without much rest. Choose 2–3 exercises per muscle group and do 2–4 sets each.

## Sample opposing muscle groups schedule

Day 1: chest, back, shoulders, abs
Day 2: off
Day 3: quads, hamstrings, calves
Day 4: off
Day 5: biceps, triceps, abs
Day 6: off
Day 7: off

### ➲ ROUTINE: push/pull

**Frequency:** 2–4-day split
**Best for:** intermediate, advanced

Similar in difficulty to the upper/lower split, the push/pull split pairs muscle groups that perform similar motions into either two or three days and is performed over 2–4 days per week. The pushing muscles include chest, shoulders, triceps, quads and calves. The pulling muscles include the back, biceps, hamstrings and abs. Choose 2–3 exercises for each muscle group and do 2–4 sets each. One major benefit of this split is that all pushing exercises are done in one day and they rest on all the other days. The push/pull philosophy can be put into action in the following ways:

## Sample 3-day split

INTERMEDIATE

Day 1: chest, shoulders, triceps, quads and calves (push day)
Day 2: off
Day 3: back, biceps, hamstrings, abs (pull day)
Day 4: off
Day 5: repeat push day
Day 6: off
Day 7: off

**Note:** *Start the next week with the pull routine and follow the same schedule, starting each week where you left off the previous week.*

## Sample 3-day split

ADVANCED

Day 1: chest, shoulders, triceps, abs
Day 2: off
Day 3: legs (quads, hamstrings and calves)
Day 4: off
Day 5: back, biceps, abs
Day 6: off
Day 7: off

# PROGRAMMING OPTIONS

At the beginning of each subsequent chapter, you'll find programs for each bodypart: abs, arms, back, chest, glutes and legs, and shoulders. The beginner and intermediate programs are six-week progressive programs that will take you to the next level. If you're advanced, you have three workout options during your workout week. We've also included a non-gym-based program. If you've never put together a program, hit a plateau or are simply looking to get out of the box, these programs are a great way to become familiar with solid training techniques, learn intensity training techniques that are built into the intermediate and advanced programs, and shake things up a bit by adding variety to your workout. If you'd rather design your own program, there are plenty of exercises to choose from in each chapter.

## SAMPLE PROGRAMS

The various training splits in the previous section are arranged from beginner to more advanced, starting with a full-body routine. If you've been doing a full-body routine, however, and are ready for a change, try one of the two-day splits, either the upper/ower or the push/pull. If you've been following a push/pull routine, try one of the four-day splits, and so on.

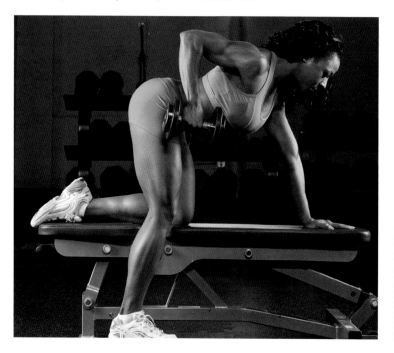

## ANSWERS TO YOUR TOP THREE QUESTIONS

*We get hundreds of letters from readers asking questions about strength training. Here are the answers to the three most common questions.*

### • *How can I get stronger without getting big and bulky?*

Don't worry about getting big. Most women simply don't have enough testosterone to develop huge muscles. In fact, most men can't even develop big muscles without working really hard at it. Female bodybuilders with masculine physiques lift extremely heavy weights for several hours a day. They also have extremely low bodyfat levels (which they can't sustain after contests) so their muscles appear even larger.

### • *Why did I gain more strength when I was a beginner than I do now?*

It wasn't because your muscles suddenly got stronger; your muscle fibers don't actually grow much in the first six weeks or so. Novice lifters tend to make dramatic gains primarily because they become more skilled and coordinated. Think about it: The first time you try the dumbbell shoulder press, you waste a lot of energy trying to keep the weights steady and move them in a relatively straight line. But once you get the hang of things, you can put all your energy into lifting the dumbbells. Meanwhile, your nerves — the pathways that link our brain and muscles — learn how to carry information more quickly. Once you master an exercise, your brain essentially tells your muscles, "You know what to do. Go for it."

• *How can I achieve muscle definition?*
A well-designed weight-training routine will strengthen, tone and shape your muscles, but in order to develop that "cut" look, you also need to minimize the layer of fat covering them. Weight training can contribute to fat loss by burning calories and preserving — or even boosting — your metabolism. However, to create the calorie deficit necessary for significant weight loss, it's best to combine strength training with cardiovascular exercise and smart eating habits. Remember: You need to burn more calories than you eat.

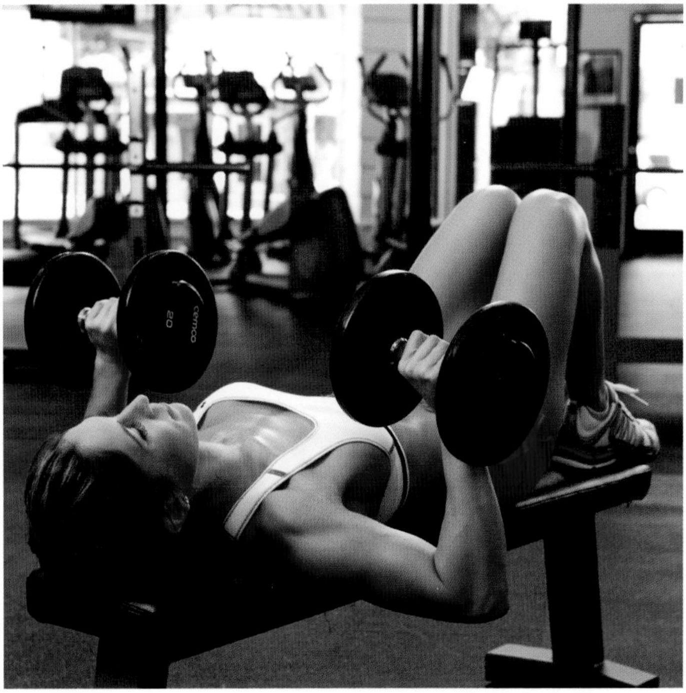

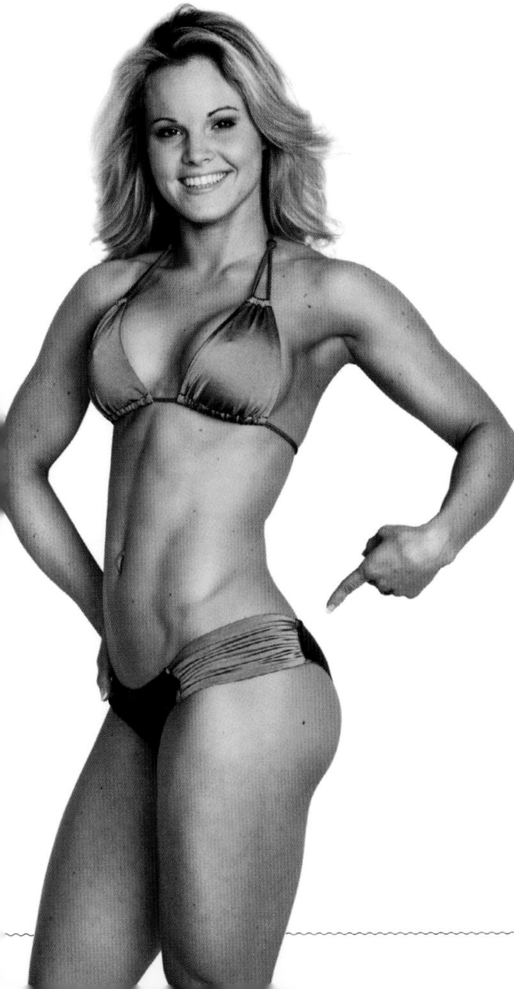

## WHERE TO GO FROM HERE

You now have much of the knowledge you need to take charge of your training program. We've condensed an enormous amount of training information into a concise, comprehensive reference and training guide that can help you achieve the results you want. The choice is now yours: You can use the pre-programmed routines listed with each bodypart, select your own exercises and plug them into these routines if you want to substitute or, if you're more advanced, try any of the high-intensity training principles or programs we've outlined for you. Regardless of your fitness experience, successful training is dependent upon consistency, trial and error, and awareness. Reps, sets, weight, exercise selection — these elements all matter. However, they are variables that will change with your goals and are sometimes less important than your attitude. The training principles and programs presented in this book are tried and true — all you need to do is find the program that fits your individual profile and your personal appeal and then just go for it. You'll be thrilled with how your body looks and feels!

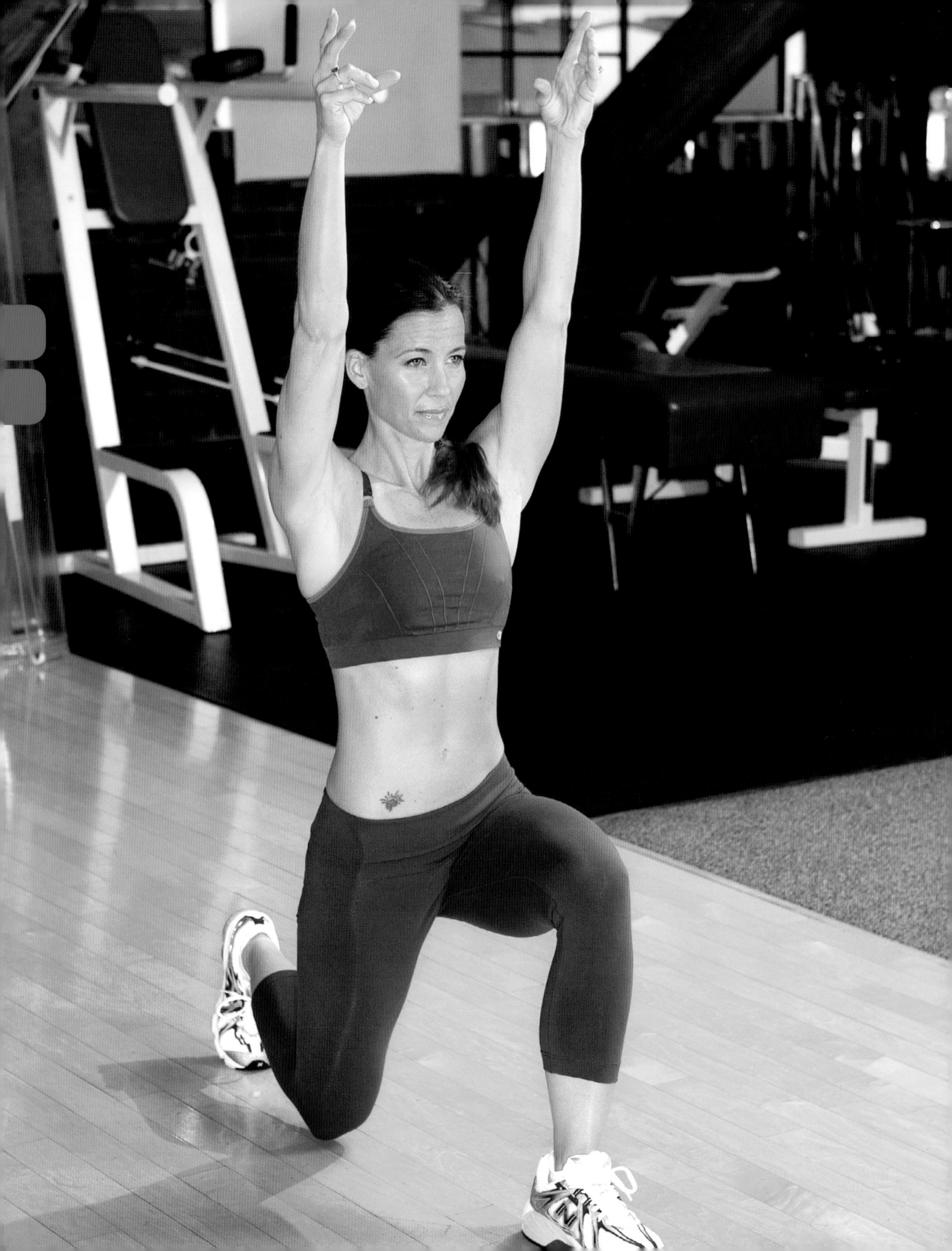

Chapter 2

# Warming Up

*A dynamic warm-up will improve your power and agility*

WARMING UP AND STRETCHING. Are these words synonymous? According to a growing body of scientific evidence, they're not. And if you're looking to improve your power and agility in the gym, you may want to add a different term to your lexicon — *dynamic warm-up*. Just as the name implies, it's not flowing movements and static poses but rather a series of calisthenics and movement drills to prepare your body for the work ahead. Recent research performed by the U.S. Army found that dynamic warm-ups increase your heart rate, body temperature, muscle and joint pliability, as well as nerve and muscle responsiveness, thus preparing your body for the tough workout ahead.

"You can use dynamic warm-ups before any fitness or sport activity, especially those that involve power and strength, such as resistance training, kick-boxing and cycling," says Michele S. Olson, PhD, CSCS, FACSM, a professor of exercise science at Auburn University in Birmingham, Alabama. "A dynamic warm-up prevents the loss of power that can occur when using static stretching as a warm-up [Ed Note: One theory suggests this happens because static stretching activates fewer motor units] and therefore reduces the likelihood of someone overdoing it to compensate for the loss of power and strength that static stretching creates."

Olson suggests that your dynamic warm-up should be specific to your workout. "Mimic the movements you're about to do using high repetitions and no weight," she says. For example, before your leg workout, do some walking lunges, high knee raises and half-squats, all without weight. "Start out slow with lower ranges, begin to increase the range of motion and then speed up the pace," Olson recommends. "This will allow your circulation to rise to keep pace with the more dynamic warm-up."

The following pages outline a dynamic warm-up routine that you can do before a full-body workout. It's based on the U.S. Army research mentioned earlier. Keep your intensity level to a low-to-moderate level to prevent fatigue, which can be difficult since some of these movements are just plain fun to do. Now go warm up!

# Bend and Reach

***Warms up:*** *Back, shoulders, hamstrings*

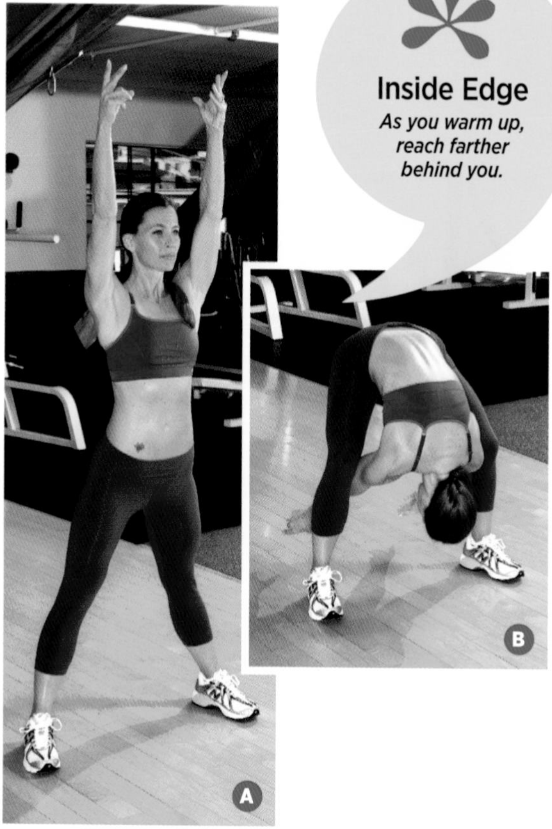

**Inside Edge**

*As you warm up, reach farther behind you.*

## Technique

1. Stand with your feet wider than shoulder-width apart and your arms reaching toward the ceiling.
2. Align your head neutrally, looking straight ahead.
3. Bend over while moving your hands forward and down in an arc so that you reach between your legs, allowing your back to flex.
4. Keep your heels on the floor.
5. Retrace your path to return to start.

**CADENCE:** Slow

## Your Dynamic Warm-Up

| EXERCISE | REPS | CADENCE |
|---|---|---|
| Bend and Reach | 10 | slow |
| Reverse Lunge and Reach | 10 | slow |
| Turn and Reach | 10 | slow |
| Sit-Up with Knee In | 10 | slow to moderate |
| Jump Squat (not shown) | 10 | moderate |
| Lying Back Extension | 10 | slow to moderate |
| Push-Up (not shown) | 10 | moderate to fast |
| Windmill | 10 | moderate to fast |
| Skip | 10 | moderate to fast |
| High Knee Raise | 10 | moderate to fast |
| Sidestep | 10 each side | moderate |

# Reverse Lunge and Reach

***Warms Up:*** *Shoulders, glutes, quadriceps, hamstrings*

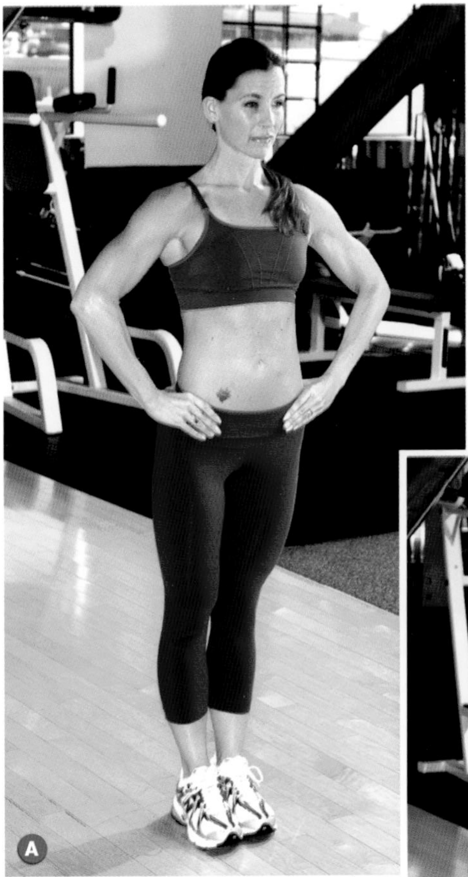


## Technique

1. Stand with your hands on your hips and your feet together.
2. Step back with one leg and plant your toes on the floor.
3. Lower yourself by bending both legs.
4. Keep most of the weight on your front leg and, at the same time, reach overhead.
5. Return to the start in one motion.

**CADENCE:** Slow

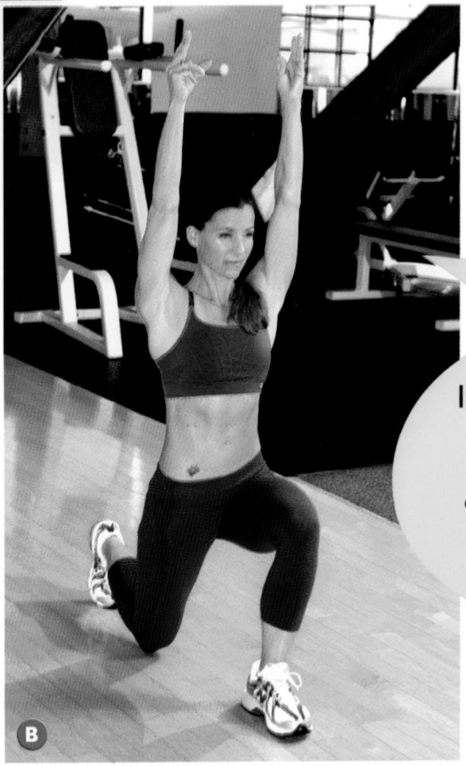


**Inside Edge**

***Lunge progressively deeper with each repetition.***

# Turn and Reach

***Warms Up:*** *Abdominals, obliques, back*

## Technique

1. Stand with your feet shoulder-width apart, arms at shoulder level and straight out to your sides, with your palms up.
2. Look straight ahead.
3. Keep your abs tight.
4. Without moving your head, hips or feet, turn your shoulders to one side with one arm forward and the other rearward.
5. Pause and return to start.
6. Repeat in opposite direction.

**CADENCE:** Slow

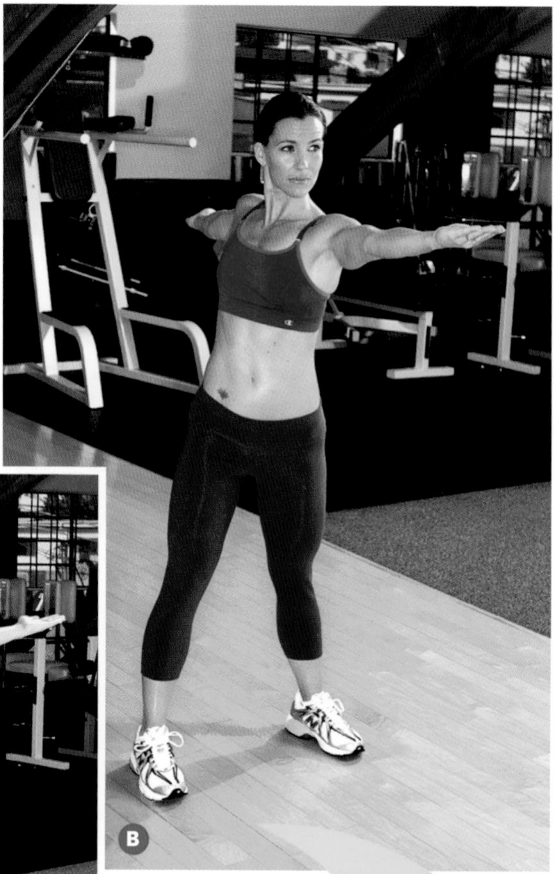

B

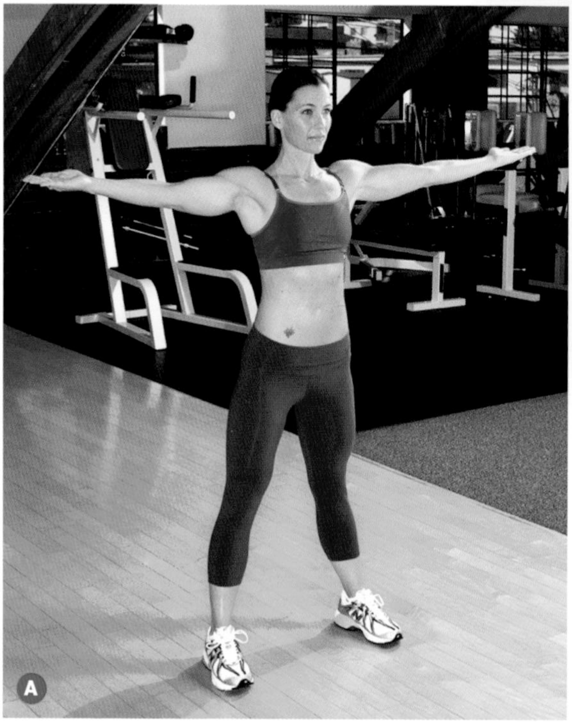

A

**Inside Edge**

***Rotate only your torso.***

# Sit-Up with Knee In

***Warms Up:*** *Abs*

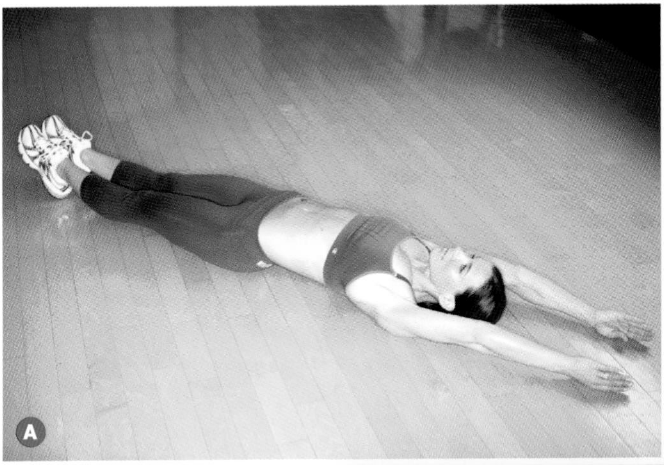

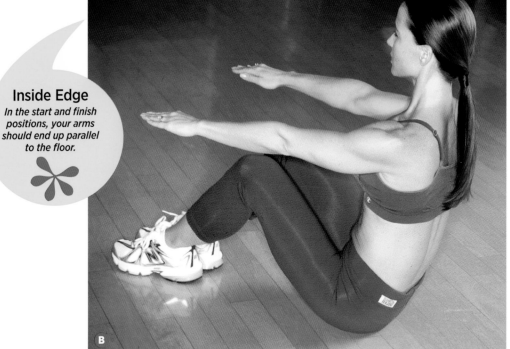


## Technique

1. Lie faceup on the floor with your arms straight overhead and your legs straight.
2. Hold your head a few inches off the floor.
3. In one motion, raise yourself to a seated position while also bending your legs until your feet are flat on the floor.
4. In the top position, your arms should be parallel to the floor.

**CADENCE:** Slow to moderate

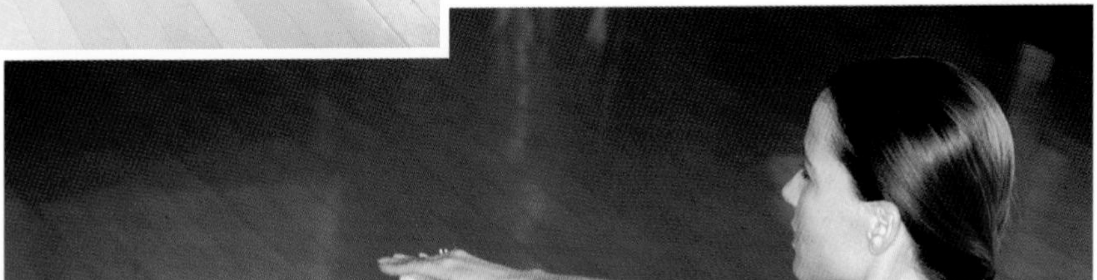


**Inside Edge**

*In the start and finish positions, your arms should end up parallel to the floor.*

# Lying Back Extension

***Warms Up:*** *Back, shoulders*

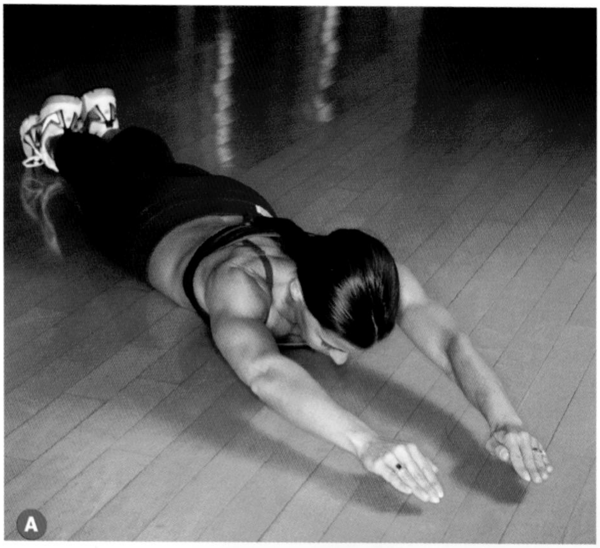


## Technique

1. Lie facedown with your arms overhead and a few inches off the floor.
2. Keep your head in a neutral position and your abs tight.
3. Raise your chest off the floor while moving your arms to shoulder level as if you're flying.
4. Return to the start position.

**CADENCE:** Slow to moderate

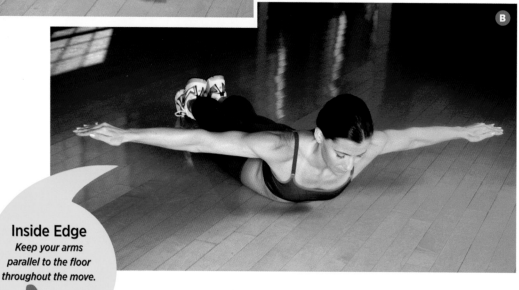


**Inside Edge**
***Keep your arms parallel to the floor throughout the move.***

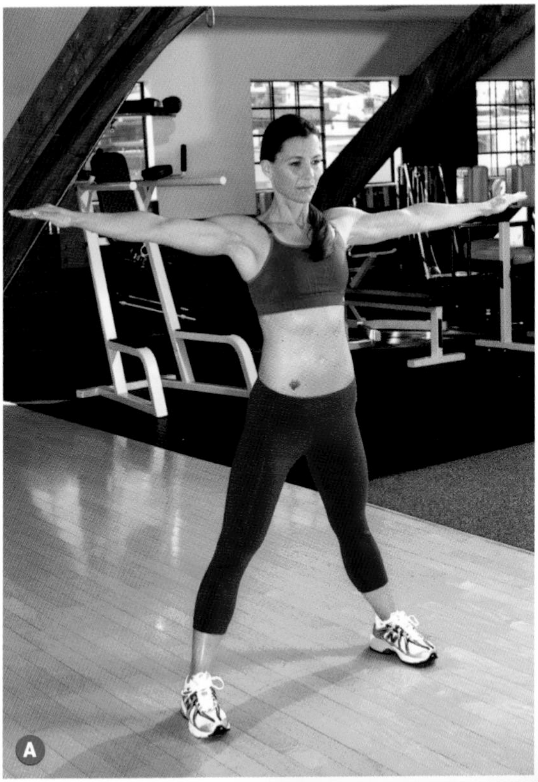


# Windmill

***Warms Up:*** *Abdominals, obliques, back*

## Technique

1. Stand in a wide stance with your arms extended in line with your shoulders.
2. Keep your head neutrally positioned and your abs tight.
3. Bend your hips and reach your right hand toward your left foot.
4. Keep your arms straight.
5. Return to the start, then repeat on your other side.

**CADENCE:** Moderate to fast

**Inside Edge**

*Be careful not to overextend your back when returning to the start.*

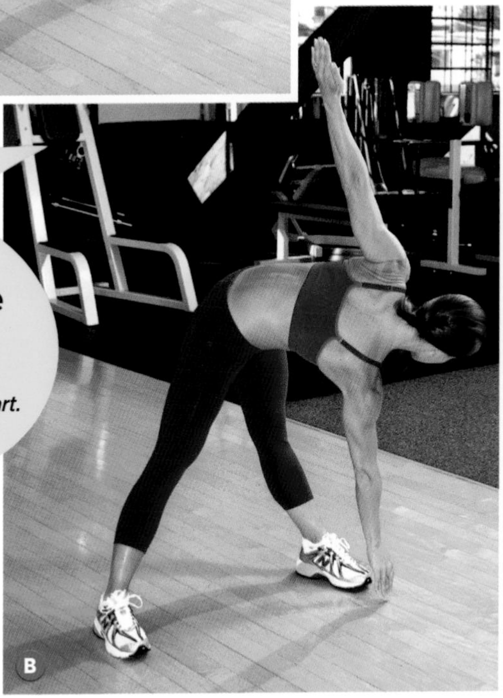


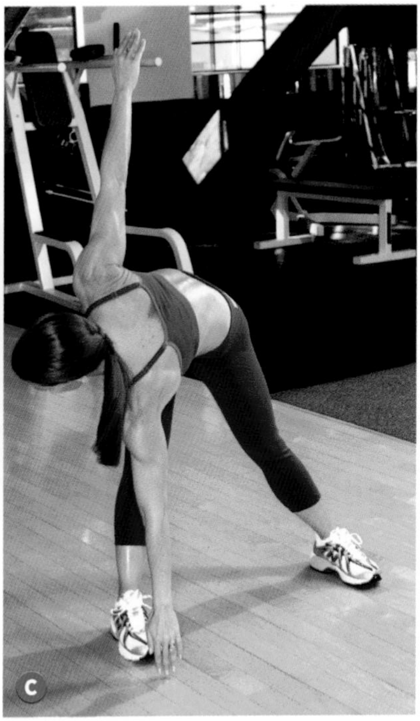

# Skip

***Warms Up:** Total body*

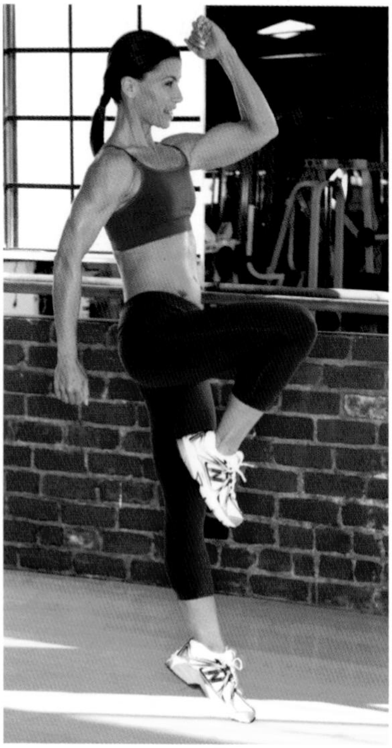

## Technique

1. Stand with your feet shoulder-width apart.
2. Keep your abs tight.
3. Step and hop, landing on the same leg that propelled you upward.
4. Now repeat with the other leg. With your arms at 90-degree angles, move them back and forth between your waist and chin, and in opposition to your legs.

**CADENCE:** Moderate to fast

**Inside Edge**

***Don't swing your legs backward — move them forward and up.***

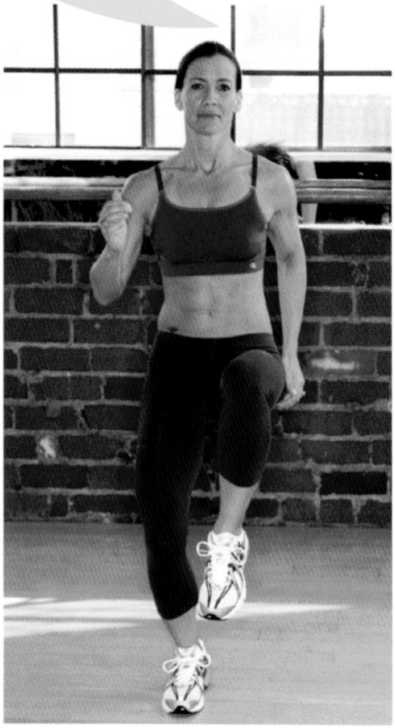

# High Knee Raise

***Warms Up:** Total body*

## Technique

1. Run forward on the balls of your feet for 10 steps.
2. Bring your knees waist high and maintain a tall stance.
3. Pump with your arms, moving them back and forth between your waist and chin.

**CADENCE:** Moderate to fast

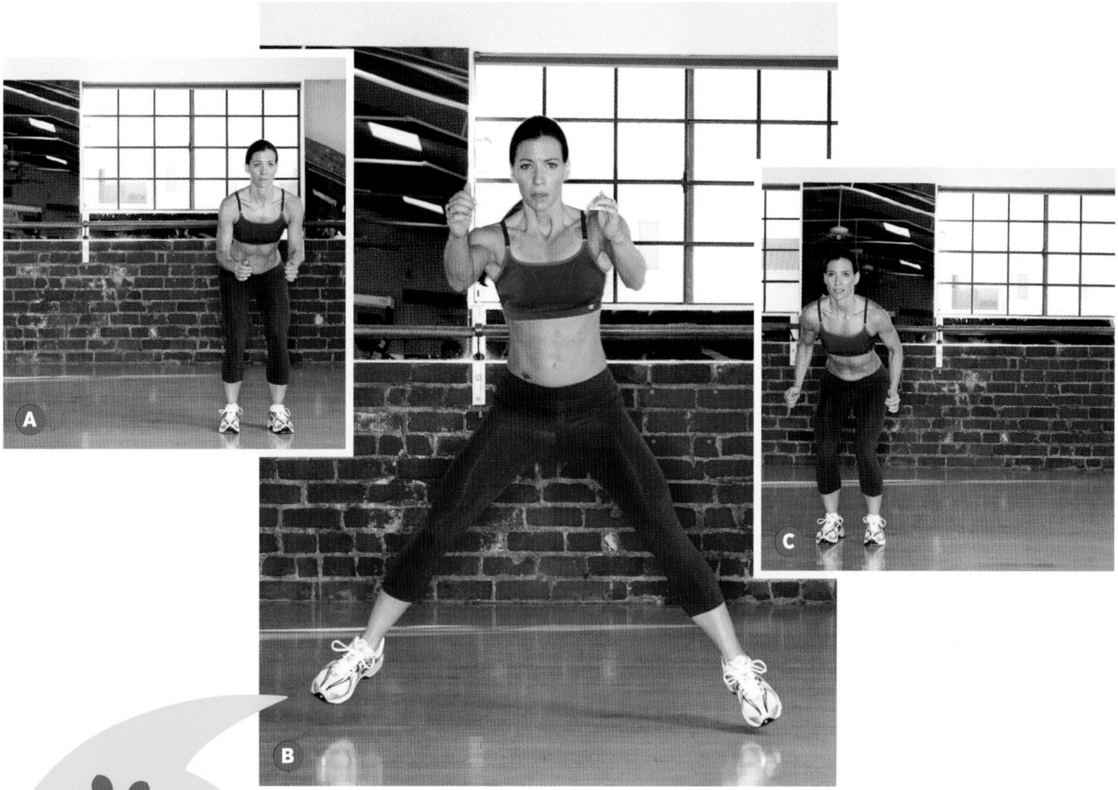


**Inside Edge**

***Keep your feet close to the floor at first, then hop progressively higher.***

# Sidestep

***Warms Up:*** *Abductors, adductors, quadriceps, hamstrings, glutes, calves*

## Technique

1. Stand in a crouched position with your back straight, abs tight and head in a neutral position looking forward.
2. Raise your torso slightly and hop to the side, bringing your trailing leg to your lead leg and landing in a crouched position.
3. Move side to side for reps.

**CADENCE:** Moderate

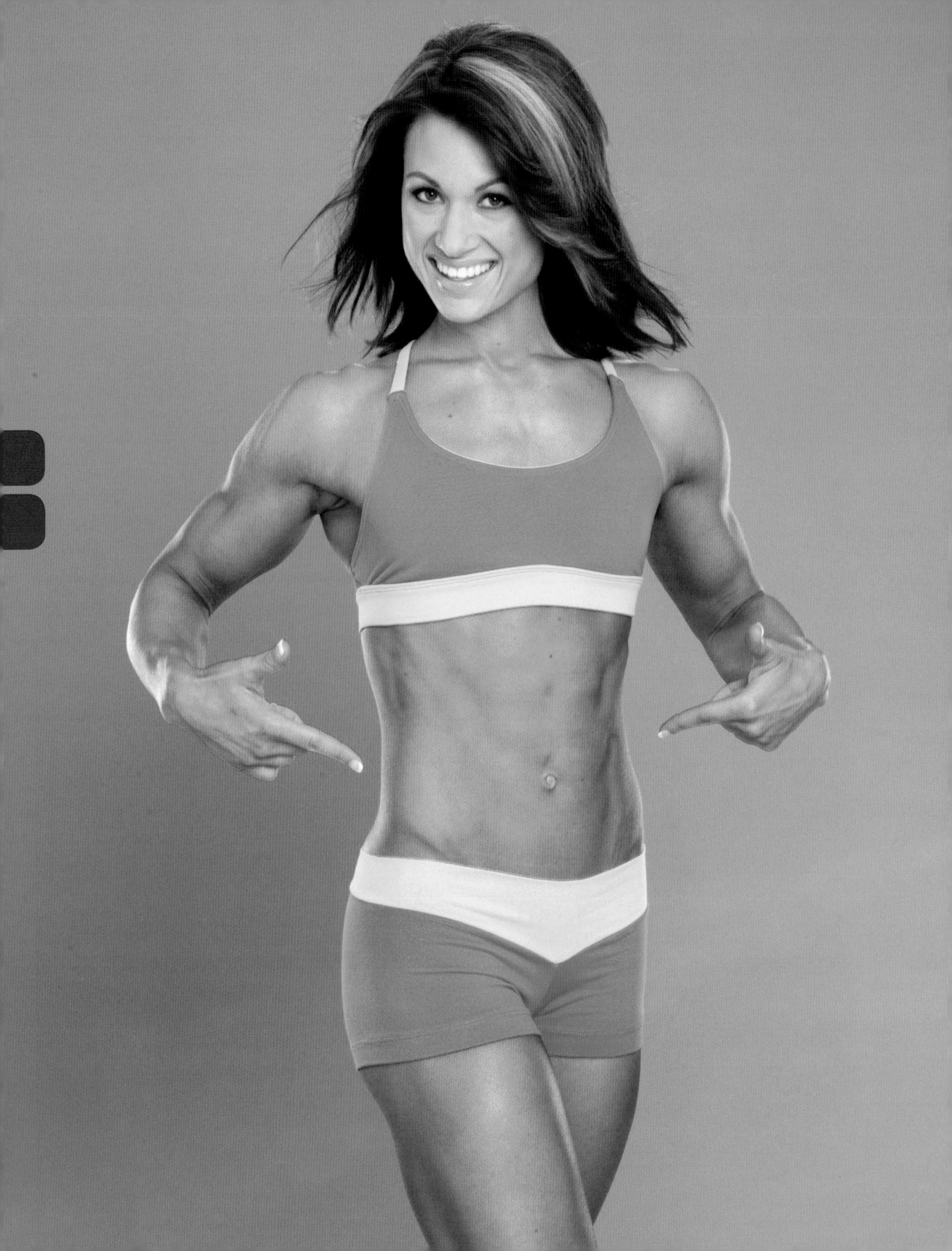

Chapter 3

# Abdominals

*Sculpt a strong midsection by working your abs from the inside out.*

THE ABDOMINALS ARE COMPRISED of four muscle groups: rectus abdominis, external obliques, internal obliques and transverse abdominis. The rectus abdominis runs from the top of the pubic bone to the sternum and flexes the torso. Attached to the connective tissue of the rectus abdominis are the external obliques, running diagonally downward from the lower ribs to the midportion of the upper pelvis bone. The internal obliques run diagonally upward from the pelvis to the lower ribs. Both oblique groups work with the rectus abdominis to flex, unilaterally rotate and laterally flex the torso. The transverse abdominis, a deep muscle running from back to front, attaches to the lower five ribs and connective tissue close to the lower spine, then runs horizontally to attach to connective tissue of the rectus abdominis. It contracts when the other abdominal muscles are working but can't be isolated. The abdominals work both as primary movers and stabilizers of the spine; it's important to include both movement types in your workout. Stabilization exercises engage the bilateral contraction of the obliques, contributing to the layering effect of the abs and forcing the transverse abdominis to support the abdominal wall and spine simultaneously as you perform each exercise repetition.

## General Guidelines for *TRAINING ABS*

Do an assortment of exercises to ensure balanced abs development, and to hit all the muscle fiber angles; no single abs exercise is perfect.

Mix up the order in which you perform exercises to continue stimulating the muscles.

Train for stabilization as well as movement, which promotes muscle endurance and forces you to maintain alignment as you move.

Vary rep speeds as well as training angles (incline, decline, flat) to manipulate the intensity and change the emphasis.

Use a variety of tools (e.g., stability balls, medicine balls) to add challenge and diversity to your program.

Complement abs work with back extensions, which stretch the front torso as you strengthen your back.

Add enough weight to fatigue your muscles, but not so much that you compromise your form.

# Ball Crunch BEGINNER

***Muscles Worked:*** *rectus abdominis, with emphasis on upper rectus fibers; external and internal obliques; transverse abdominis*

## Technique

1. Sitting upright on a stability ball, walk feet out in front of you, letting ball roll up your spine. Your torso, from shoulder blades to hips, is supported by the ball at a slight incline.
2. Keep your feet flat on floor, knees bent at 90 degrees and in line with ankles.
3. Place hands unclasped behind head or fold arms across chest, hands on opposite shoulders.
4. Contracting your abdominal muscles to bring spine to a neutral position, tuck your chin in slightly and focus on a spot straight ahead.
5. Curl torso upward, moving as one unit, only flexing from the spine.
6. Pause, then lower to start position.

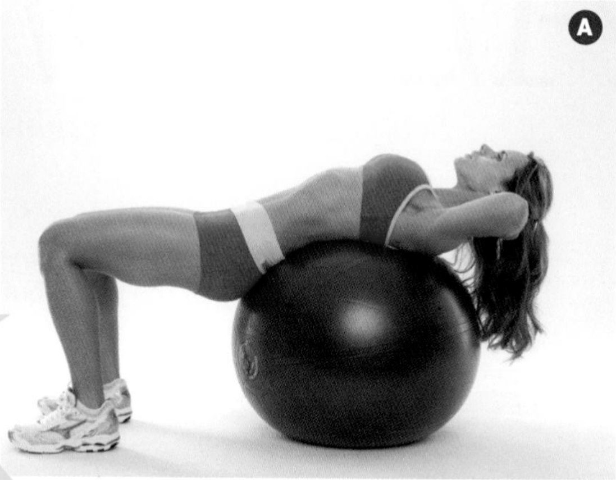


### Inside Edge

***Keeping glutes relaxed, "set" your position before crunching, bringing ribs to hips; this will fully engage your abs and control your range of motion.***

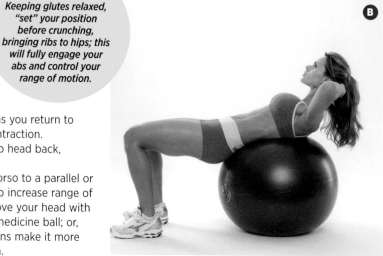

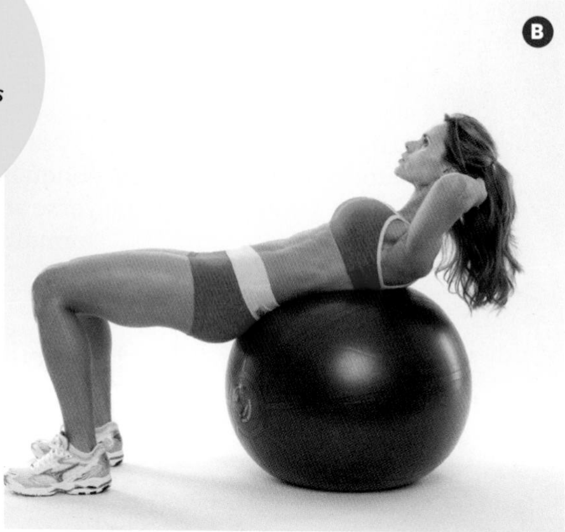


## Trainer's tips

- Keep tension on abs throughout the entire range of motion; continue to curl torso upward until the abs have reached full contraction.
- Don't release and relax the abs as you return to the start position; maintain a contraction.
- Don't press head forward or drop head back, which can cause neck strain.
- For more of a challenge, lower torso to a parallel or slightly-below-parallel position to increase range of motion; place hands or arms above your head with or without resistance such as a medicine ball; or, walk feet forward. These variations make it more difficult to stabilize your position.

# Ball Pike ADVANCED

***Muscles Worked:*** *rectus abdominis, with emphasis on lower fibers; external and internal obliques; transverse abdominis*

## Technique

1. Drape yourself facedown on a stability ball, then use your hands to slowly walk yourself forward until your shins and ankles are resting on the ball. Arms are straight, shoulders in line with wrists and body forms one straight line from head to hips in "plank."
2. Contract your abdominal muscles to support your spine.
3. Exhale and, keeping head neutral, draw legs up so that your body forms an inverted V with feet pressing against the ball as it rolls toward you.
4. Inhale and roll ball back by slowly rolling the ball to bring your legs back to plank, keeping your abs contracted and your back in a neutral position.

## Performance

- Use your abs, not your legs, to roll the ball toward you, taking you up into the pike position.
- As you move into the pike, don't shoot your shoulders past your wrists; this can cause you to lose balance as well as strain shoulder, wrist and neck muscles.
- Maintain a perfect plank and return to this position each time without letting your belly sag.
- Keep head and neck aligned with your spine, both in plank and pike.
- From the pike position, use your abs to roll the ball back out to the start position.
- For an easier version, do the Plank-to-Knee Tuck (page 42).

**Inside Edge**

***Imagine a string wrapped around your hips like a sling; it lifts you into a pike as your navel draws in toward your spine.***

A

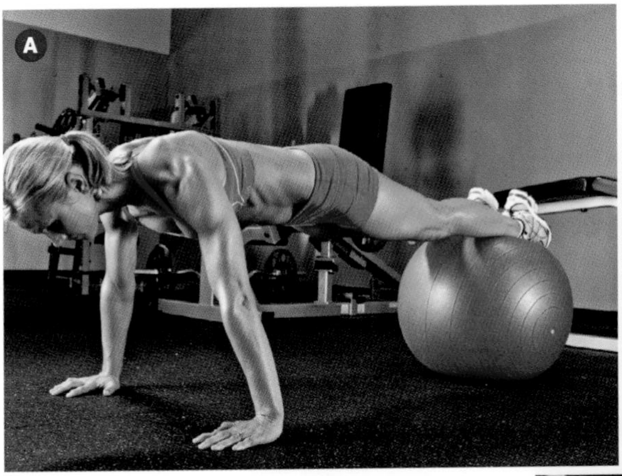

B

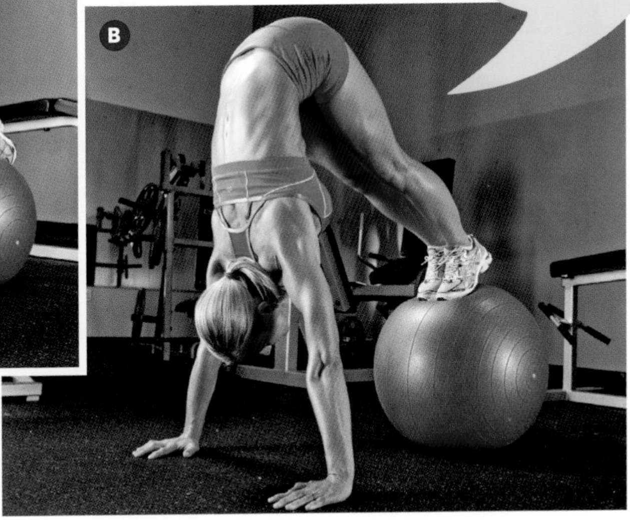

# Cross-Body Crunch

BEGINNER/INTERMEDIATE

***Muscles Worked:*** *external and internal obliques, rectus abdominis, transverse abdominis*

## Technique

1. Lie faceup on the floor, and place your fingertips unclasped behind your head. Knees are bent and in line with ankles, feet flat on the floor.
2. Contract your abdominal muscles, bringing lower hips and ribs together so spine is in a neutral position, glutes relaxed.
3. Slowly lift your torso up, head, neck and shoulder blades off the floor as you simultaneously lift one foot off the floor, bending knee in and toward your chest. Rotate your opposite shoulder toward the lifted knee by the end of the motion.
4. Slowly uncurl, lowering upper torso and leg to start position and repeat, alternating opposite elbow and knee.

## Trainer's tips

- Lift torso before you rotate; this will stimulate all of your abdominal muscle fibers and keep your torso from rolling from side to side.
- As you lift your foot, bring knee directly in toward your chest, keeping hips square and firmly on the floor.
- Keep elbow open, shoulder and armpit aimed toward opposite knee.
- Make the lift and rotation a smooth, not segmented action.
- Don't rock hips from side to side as you change legs; this decreases stabilization.
- To increase the challenge, straighten the leg in the air once the opposite knee is bent and in line with hip. Then, bend knee to lower.

### Inside Edge

***Once lifted, rotate the torso as one unit. The amount of rotation depends on your ability to contract the opposite external oblique while stabilizing your position.***

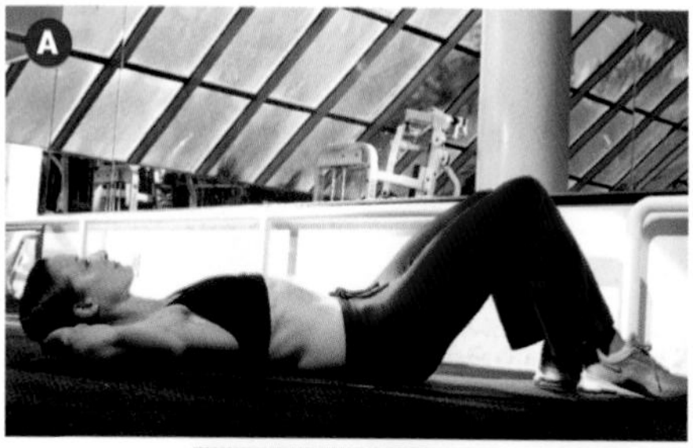
A

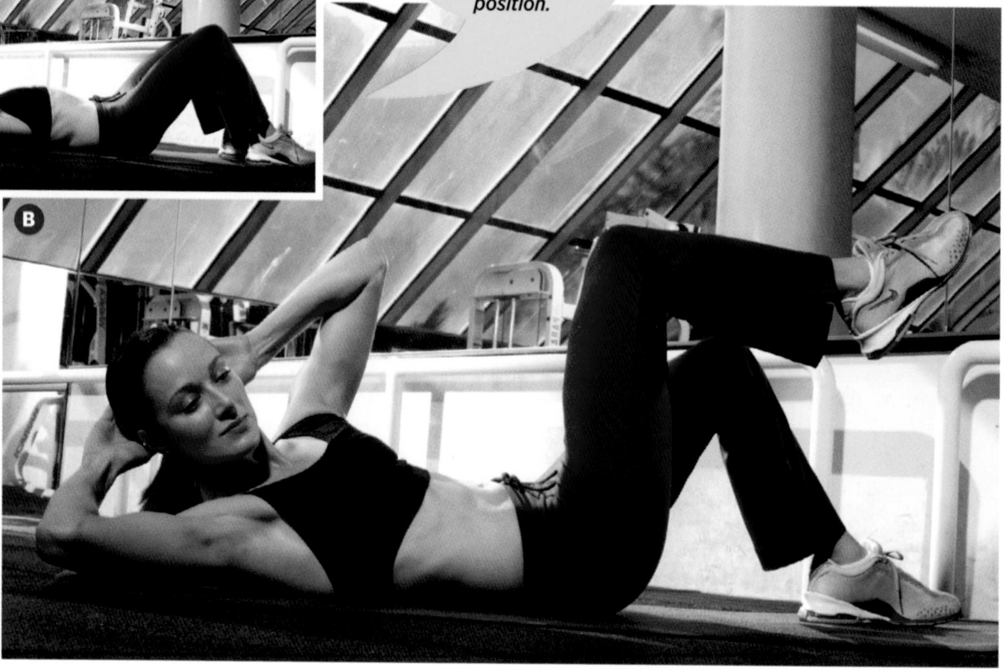
B

# Decline Weighted Twist ADVANCED

***Muscles Worked:*** *external and internal obliques; rectus abdominis and transverse abdominis as stabilizers*

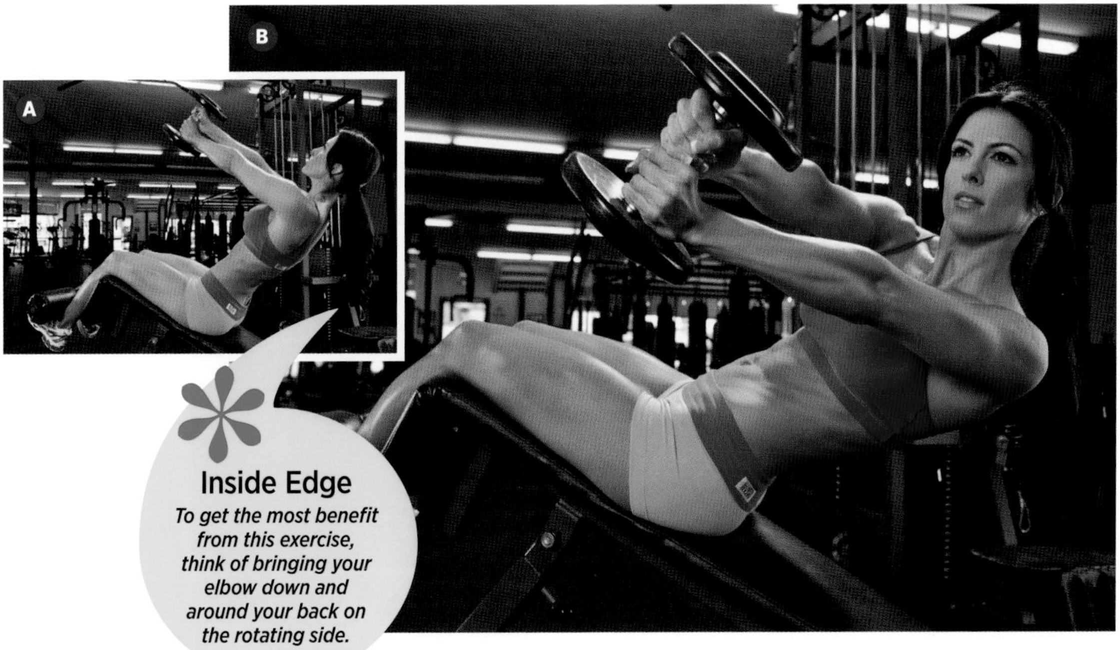


**Inside Edge**

***To get the most benefit from this exercise, think of bringing your elbow down and around your back on the rotating side.***

## Technique

1. Grasp a dumbbell, weight plate or medicine ball and sit upright on the high side of a decline bench, feet secured under footpads.
2. Contract abdominal muscles, bringing hips and lower ribs together. Keeping abs contracted to stabilize position, lean back from your hips until your torso is at a 45- to 60-degree angle to the bench.
3. Holding the weight with both hands in front of your upper rib cage, elbows bent, gently rotate torso to the right, then come back through center and rotate to the left.
4. Continue to alternate from side to side, staying lifted and erect, keeping constant tension on your abs.

## Trainer's tips

- Maintain an erect torso even though you are leaning back; stay lifted as you rotate from side to side.
- Keep elbows bent and close to your sides; don't hold the ball so far out in front of you that you strain your shoulders and back.
- Don't lean back so far that you feel a strain in your lower back.
- Continue to pull your abs up and in, with chest open and shoulder blades drawn down and together.
- Use slow, controlled movement as opposed to quick twisting.
- For variety, do this exercise seated on a stability ball and inclined, with feet flat on the floor.

# Half Rollback on Ball BEGINNER

***Muscles Worked:** rectus abdominis, external and internal obliques, transverse abdominis*

## Technique

1. Sit erect on a stability ball with knees bent, feet flat on floor and separated just wider than hip-width apart.
2. Cross forearms in front of you at chest height, squeezing shoulder blades down and together.
3. Contract abdominal muscles without collapsing torso, and tilt pelvis to stabilize your position. Continue to contract abs to roll backwards on the ball.
4. In the final position, your mid-back and spine will be in contact with the ball, abs fully contracted.
5. Keeping abs contracted, curl ribs toward pelvis to roll back up to an erect sitting position.

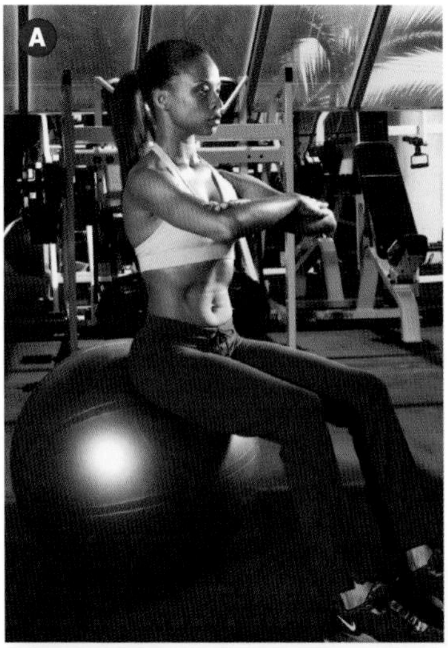


## Trainer's tips

- Let your abs do the work; don't push yourself back with your feet.
- As you return to start position, "roll" up and then extend your spine at the top, stacking shoulders in a direct line over hips.
- Move slowly with each rep. Exhale as you roll back, and inhale as you roll up.
- Keep your chin level; don't tuck or lift your chin as you roll.
- Maintain the pelvic tilt to stabilize your position on the ball.
- To make the exercise more challenging, follow this progression: Place unclasped fingertips behind head, extend arms overhead, hold a weight over your chest.

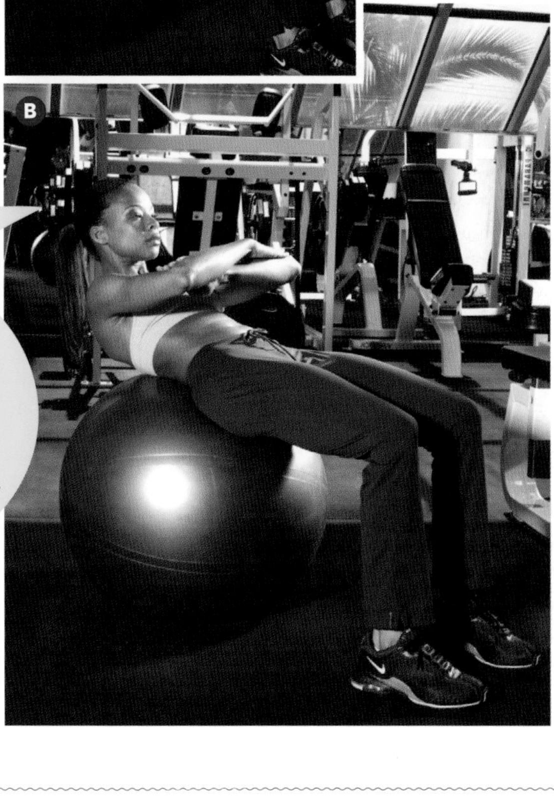


**Inside Edge**

***Keep your spine rounded rather than straight as you lower. This engages your abs rather than hip flexors and also protects your spine.***

# Hanging Leg Raise ADVANCED

***Muscles Worked:*** *rectus abdominis, with emphasis on lower fibers, internal obliques, external obliques, transverse abdominis*

## Technique

1. Find a pull-up bar at a cable station or Smith machine. Place a box or bench on the floor under the bar to help you get into position.
2. Grab onto the pull-up bar with an overhand grip, hands about shoulder-width apart.
3. Hanging with legs straight and together, bend and lift knees until thighs are parallel to floor, ankles in line with knees.
4. Without swinging, keep legs bent and curl pelvis upward in a reverse curl, drawing navel to spine.
5. Continue to curl upward until abs feel fully contracted.
6. Pause, then slowly lower your legs to the start position.

## Trainer's tips

- If you tend to swing or kick your legs up, have a spotter place her hand on your lower back to assist you in holding the position.
- Keep your torso straight, and shoulder blades drawn down and together without rounding upper back; doing so can strain your shoulders and also minimizes the exercise's efficiency.
- Don't curl your pelvis upward until your thighs have reached the lifted and parallel position, otherwise it will be too difficult to perform this latter part of the movement.
- For variety, do the same exercise using a roman chair.

**Inside Edge**

***Focus on using your abs to both lift your legs and perform the reverse curl using a slow, controlled movement.***

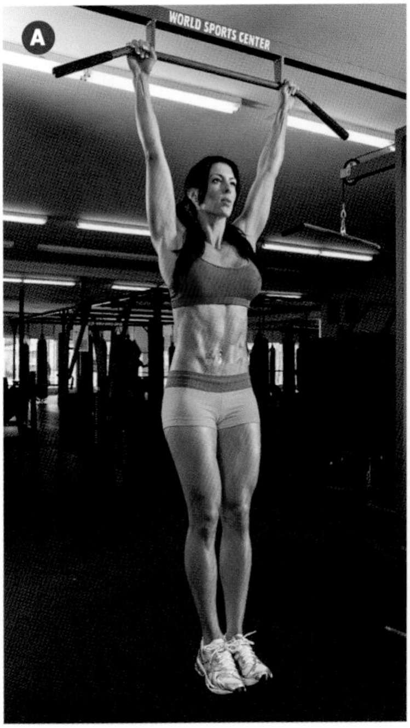


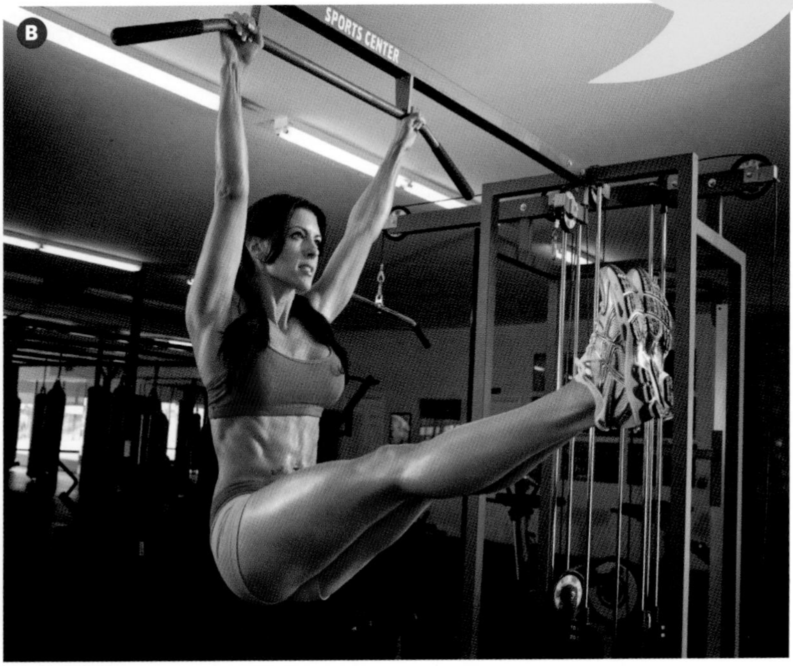

# High-Cable Chop INTERMEDIATE

***Muscles Worked:** external and internal obliques, upper fibers of rectus abdominis, transverse abdominis, lower fibers of rectus abdominis as stabilizers*

## Technique

1. Attach a single handle to a high-cable pulley, then stand with your left side to the machine at a slight diagonal. Take one large step away from machine and stand with your feet hip-width apart, knees slightly bent, and toes pointing at an angle.
2. Hold the handle with both hands, keeping hips and shoulders square.
3. Maintain position and pull handle down and toward the outside of your right hip, letting torso follow the movement, but keeping feet flat and hips square so all movement initiates from your torso.
4. Control the movement, keeping abdominal muscles contracted as you return to start position.
5. Do all reps, then switch sides.

## Trainer's tips

- Don't swing the cable handle down as if you were swinging a golf club; rotate slowly from your center without twisting hips.
- Keep your shoulders relaxed and don't pull down just by using your arms; keep your abs actively engaged throughout the entire range of motion.
- First contract your abs, then rotate; this will engage all of your abdominal muscles to fire responsively.
- For variety, do this move using a rope, or try attaching a handle to the lower cable and perform the same movement, rotating from low to high.

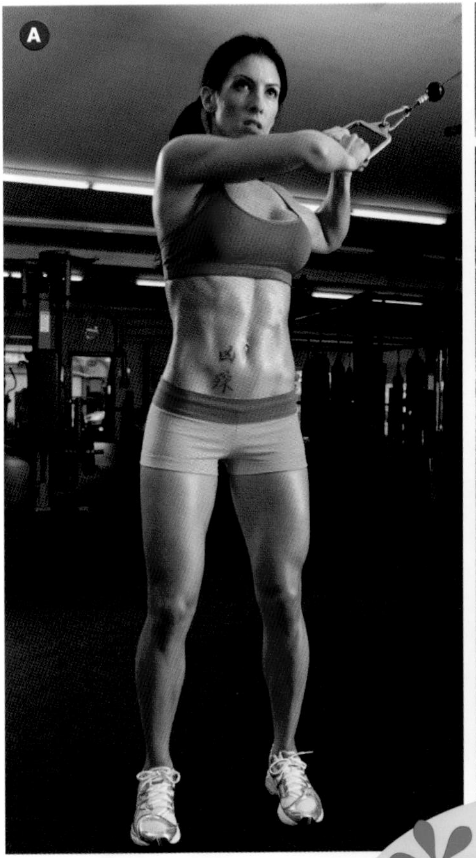


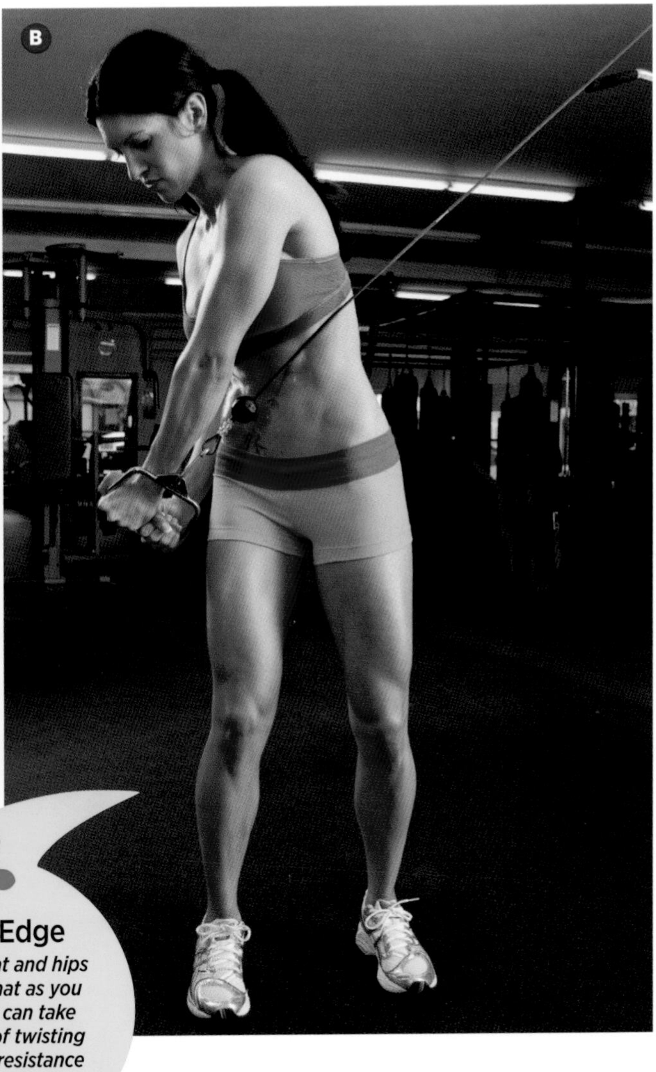


**Inside Edge**

*Keep feet flat and hips square so that as you rotate, you can take advantage of twisting against the resistance of a stable lower body.*

# Hip Thrust INTERMEDIATE/ADVANCED

***Muscles Worked:*** *rectus abdominis, with emphasis on lower fibers; transverse abdominis; external and internal obliques act as stabilizers*

## Technique

1. Lie faceup on the floor with your legs straight up in the air and in line with your hips. Grasp a bench or other stable piece of equipment with your arms straight back behind your head, shoulders relaxed and in contact with the floor, chest open.
2. Contract your abdominal muscles, bringing lower ribs and hips toward each other so your spine is in a neutral position; allow tailbone to rest on the floor, glutes relaxed.
3. Inhale, then exhale, using abs to lift hips a few inches off the floor, pressing feet upward toward the ceiling.
4. Pause for 1–2 seconds, then lower hips to the floor without changing leg position.

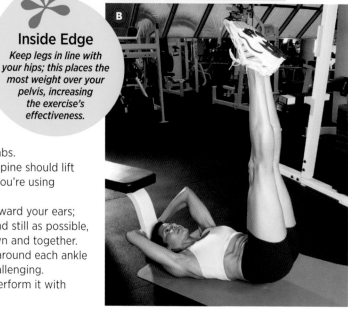

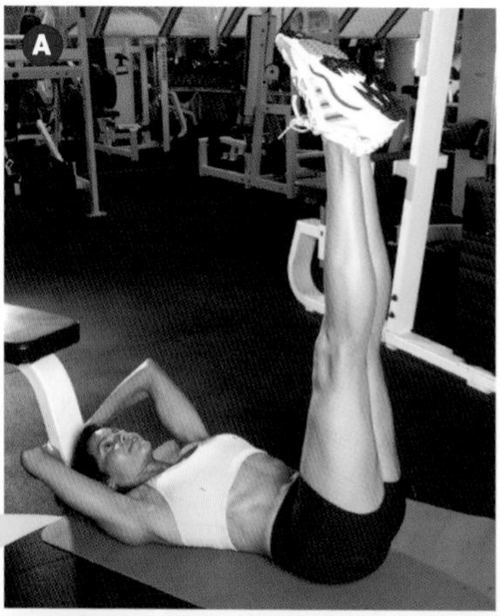


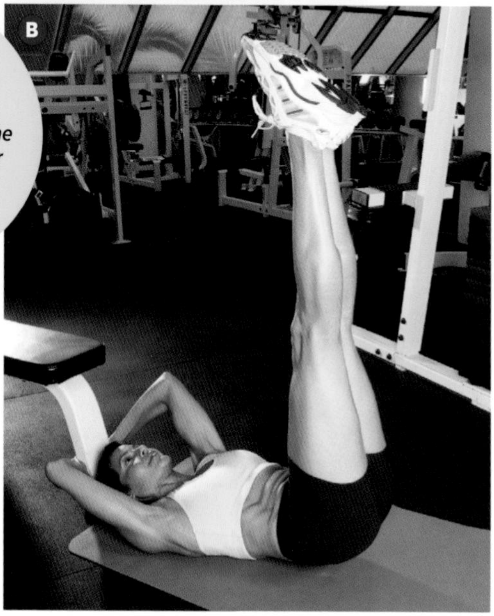


**Inside Edge**

***Keep legs in line with your hips; this places the most weight over your pelvis, increasing the exercise's effectiveness.***

## Trainer's tips

- Imagine keeping your legs motionless and vertical as you lift and lower. They shouldn't waver toward your head or drop toward the floor; all of the action comes from the contraction of your abs.
- Only your tailbone and lower spine should lift off the floor; any higher and you're using momentum.
- Don't hunch your shoulders toward your ears; keep upper torso as relaxed and still as possible, shoulder blades squeezed down and together.
- Place a 2- to 5-pound weight around each ankle to make this exercise more challenging.
- To make this exercise easier, perform it with knees bent.

# Leg and Arm Press BEGINNER/INTERMEDIATE

***Muscles Worked:*** *abdominals, with emphasis on deep transverse contraction and bilateral contraction of the obliques*

## Technique

1. Lie faceup on the floor with legs lifted, knees bent at 90-degree angles and aligned with hips, calves parallel to the floor.
2. Extend arms in the air so they're aligned directly over your shoulders, palms facing forward.
3. Tighten your abdominal muscles, closing ribs and hips together to stabilize spine.
4. Keeping abs contracted, exhale and extend both legs to a 45-degree angle while simultaneously lowering both arms behind your head, toward the floor.
5. As you extend your legs, the angles in your knees and hips will increase, but straighten your legs only as far as you can without arching your back.
6. Return to start position.

## Trainer's tips

- Keep your chin level and neck lengthened; the back of your head remains in contact with the floor.
- Don't let your abs "pooch" out as you extend your legs; think of keeping them flat by continuing to contract and pull them inward as you extend your legs.
- Keep your entire back in contact with the floor through both the extending and bending phases of the movement.
- Don't drop your legs lower than 45 degrees, which can stress your spine.
- For more of a challenge, do this exercise with head, neck and shoulder blades in a sustained lift off the floor for all reps.

### Inside Edge

***Using navel as center point, extend arms and legs away from each other, as if pulling them apart.***

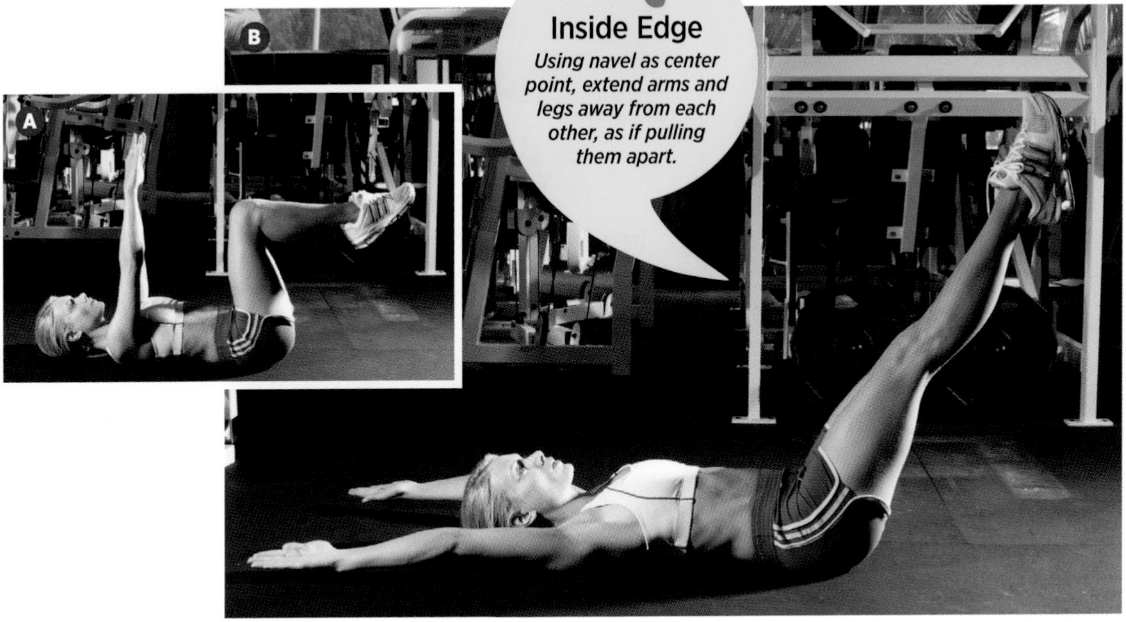

# Medicine-Ball Oblique Crunch

INTERMEDIATE/ADVANCED

***Muscles Worked:*** *rectus abdominis, with emphasis on the external and internal obliques; transverse abdominis*

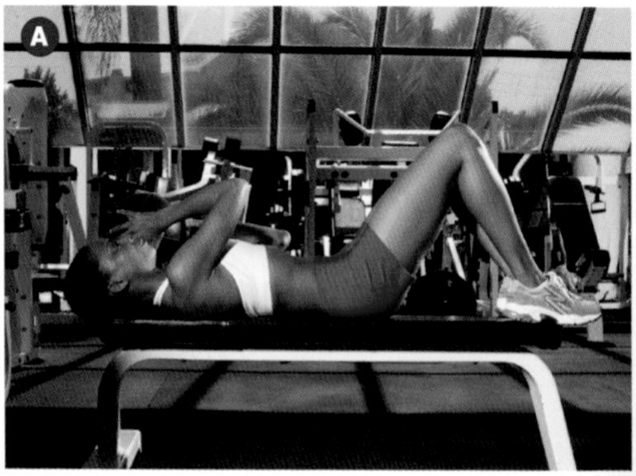


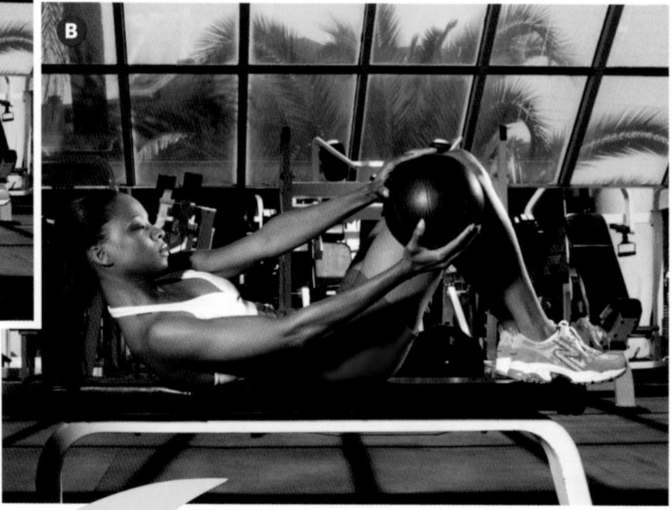


## Technique

1. Lie faceup on a flat bench, knees bent and feet on the edge of the bench. Grasp a medicine ball in both hands, then extend arms over left shoulder and up close to left ear, elbows bent.
2. Tighten abdominal muscles, drawing lower ribs and hips together to bring spine into a neutral position.
3. Contract abs to curl head, neck and shoulder blades off bench and at the same time, "chop" the ball downward, crossing arms to the outside of right knee.
4. Return to start position, using a slow, controlled motion and maintaining tension on your abs.
5. Repeat for all reps, then switch sides to complete 1 set.

### Inside Edge

***Your arms and the ball follow the rotation of your torso; this ensures the initial contraction comes from your abs.***

## Trainer's tips

- Think about lifting the torso first, then rotating as one action.
- Keep hips square and stable; the motion consistently comes from your abs.
- Be sure to exhale with the lift, inhale with the return.
- Keep head and neck relaxed, shoulders pulled down and away from your ears.
- Keep glutes relaxed, tailbone in contact with the bench.
- To make this move easier, use an incline bench instead of a flat bench.
- To increase intensity, use a decline bench.

# Medicine-Ball Reverse Crunch

INTERMEDIATE/ADVANCED

***Muscles Worked:*** *rectus abdominis, emphasizing lower fibers, transverse abdominis, internal obliques; external obliques and upper fibers of the rectus as stabilizers*

## Technique

1. Lying faceup on the floor, place a medicine ball between your knees, then grip the ball to hold it in place. Bring your knees in toward your chest and align them with your hips, calves parallel to the floor.
2. Grasp a sturdy object, such as the base of a weight bench, behind your head with both hands, elbows slightly bent.
3. Contract abdominal muscles, bringing lower ribs and hips together so spine is in a neutral position, buttocks relaxed.
4. Maintaining leg position, use your abs to curl hips a few inches off the floor.
5. Pause for two seconds, then slowly lower.

## Trainer's tips

- Avoid using a weight so heavy that you can't lift your hips off the floor; this takes the workload off your abs, and can potentially strain your back muscles.
- Don't use momentum to lift or "throw" your legs up toward your shoulders; not only is this ineffective abs training, it places stress on both your back and neck.
- Maintain control of the downward motion as you return your hips to the floor so you don't arch your back or drop your legs.
- For more of a challenge, lie on a balance tool such as a BOSU.

**Inside Edge**

***Curl your hips off the floor by bringing them up toward your ribs rather than performing a thrusting upward motion with your legs.***

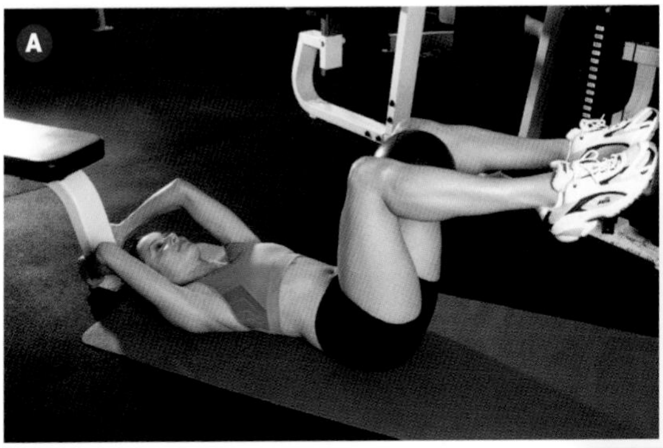
A

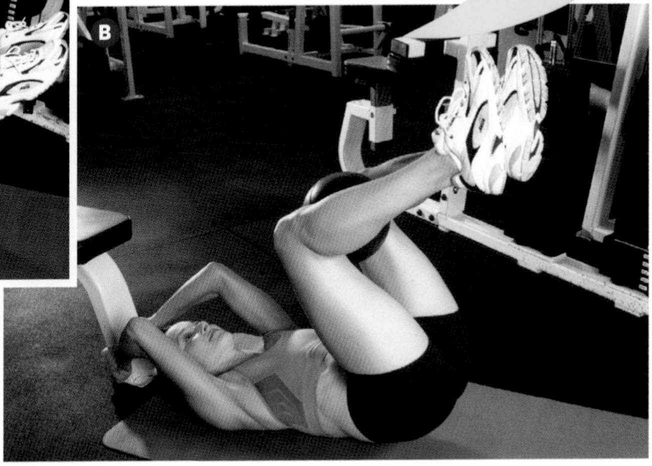
B

# Plank-to-Knee Tuck INTERMEDIATE/ADVANCED

***Muscles Worked:** rectus abdominis, with emphasis on lower fibers; bilateral contraction of external and internal obliques and transverse abdominis to stabilize torso*

## Technique

1. Drape yourself facedown on a stability ball, palms flat on floor, arms straight but not locked.
2. Slowly walk yourself forward using your hands until your shins and tops of feet are pressing on the top of the ball, arms straight, shoulders in line with wrists. Your body forms one straight line from head to hips in "plank" position.
3. Contract your abdominal muscles to support spine and prevent arching. Exhale and draw your knees toward your chest; ball rolls toward you.
4. Inhale and slowly extend your legs back to plank position, keeping your abs contracted and your back in a neutral position throughout the entire exercise.

## Trainer's tips

- Learn how to maintain a perfect plank position before attempting the tuck. Stay in plank for 30–60 seconds; if your abs can't support the position, you're not ready for the tuck.
- Keep your head and neck in a neutral position, shoulders down and away from your ears.
- As you tuck, maintain the same upper-body position so your shoulders and wrists stay aligned.
- Don't squeeze your shoulder blades together so tightly that your upper back "sinks."
- Control the ball as you straighten your legs, keeping hips level.
- For more of a challenge, try a Ball Pike (page 31).

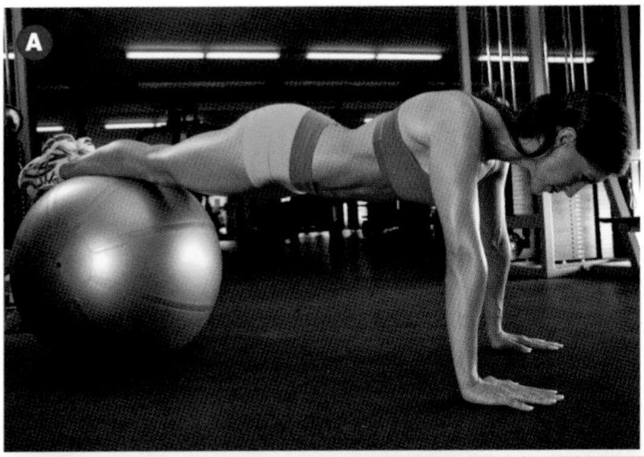


### Inside Edge

*Use your abs to initiate the movement of the ball instead of just pulling the ball toward you with your legs.*

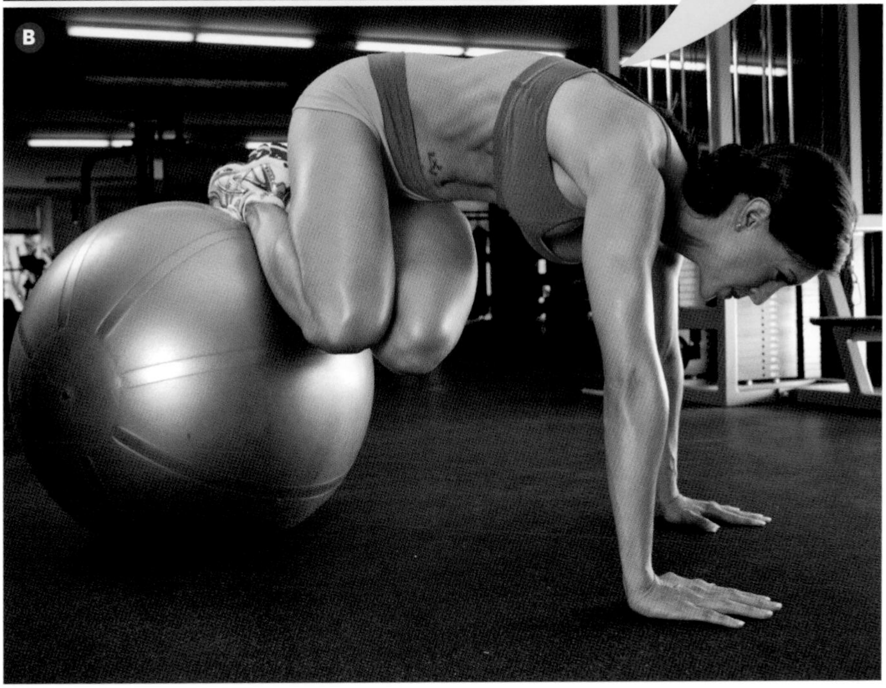

# Reverse Trunk Twist BEGINNER

***Muscles Worked:*** *external and internal obliques; lower fibers of rectus abdominis and transverse abdominis as stabilizers*

## Technique

1. Lie faceup on the floor, arms extended at shoulder height and straight out to your sides, palms down.
2. Lift your legs and bend your knees so that your knees and hips both form 90-degree angles, calves parallel to the floor, legs squeezed together.
3. Contract your abdominal muscles, bringing ribs and hips together.
4. Inhale and slowly lower your knees to one side, keeping shoulders square and on the floor. Exhale, fully contracting abs to bring legs back to center and repeat, alternating to the other side.
5. Only lower your legs as far as you can to still use your abs to bring your legs back to center.

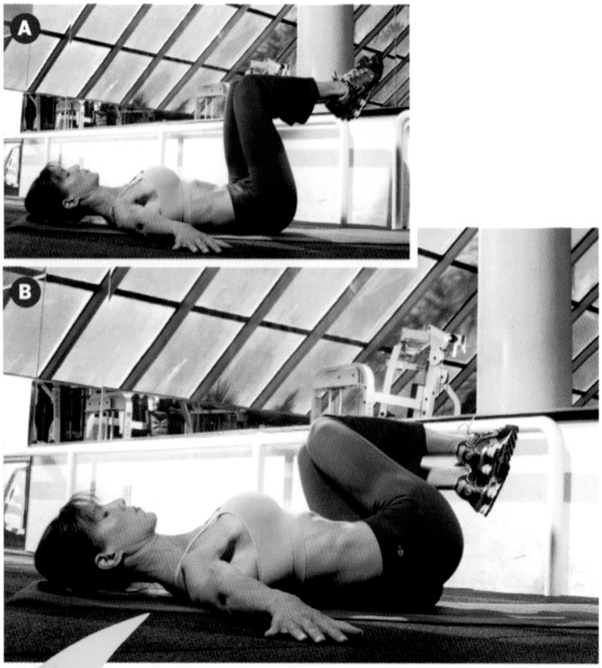


## Trainer's tips

- Keep your chin in a neutral, level position; use your thighs as a focal point.
- Keep your thighs level and motionless; they move side to side rather than in toward your chest or dropping toward your feet.
- Inhale and exhale with every rep to get deeper into your abs; without the contraction, you'll just be rolling from side to side.
- Stabilize your torso by drawing your shoulder blades down and back; this helps keep your shoulders down and relaxed on the floor as well.
- To make this exercise less challenging, bend your knees more, dropping your heels toward your buttocks.

**Inside Edge**

***Use your abs, rather than your legs, to facilitate movement. Think of your navel as your pivotal center and generate the contraction at that point.***

# Scissor Cycle

INTERMEDIATE/ADVANCED

***Muscles Worked:*** *rectus abdominis, with emphasis on the upper fibers; transverse abdominis; external and internal obliques as stabilizers*

## Technique

1. Lie faceup on the floor, with both legs together and extended in the air above your hips, palms resting between your knees and shins.
2. Contract your abdominal muscles and let your shoulder blades clear the floor. Chin is level, your lower and middle back remain firmly on the floor.
3. Lower your right leg toward the floor, keeping your right hand on that leg. At the same time, move your left arm behind you, aligned with your left ear.
4. Begin alternating, lowering your left leg and left arm as you raise your right leg (in the air) and right arm (back toward your ear). Continue this "scissor" fashion to complete the set.

## Trainer's tips

- Your same-side arm and leg should move as if they are joined by a string; when one leg lifts, the arm lifts at the same time and at the same speed; as the leg lowers, so does the arm.
- The lower your legs, the harder it is to keep your back firmly pressed into the floor.
- If your back starts lifting off the mat, you're lowering your leg too far. Your entire back should remain pressed to the floor.
- To increase intensity, reach both arms behind your head as your one leg lifts, lower arms as the other leg comes up.

**Inside Edge**

***Focus on lengthening the arm and leg away from each other as you continually compress your abs in and down toward the floor.***

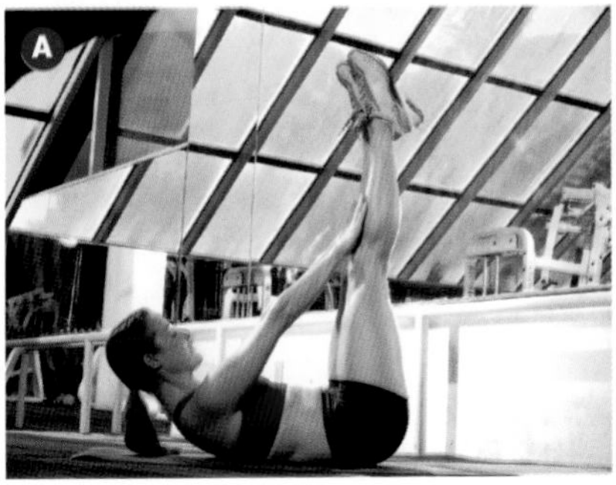


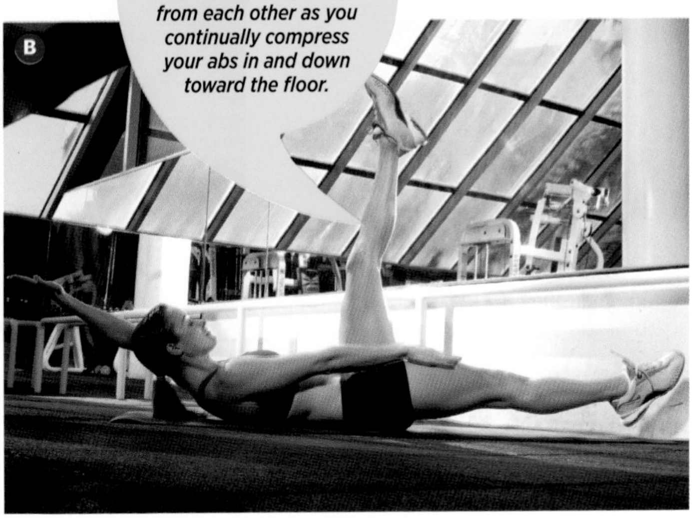

# Sidewinder INTERMEDIATE

***Muscles Worked:*** *external obliques, internal obliques, transverse abdominis; rectus abdominis as stabilizer*

## Technique

1. Lie faceup on the floor, knees bent, feet flat on the floor, head and shoulder blades raised.
2. Contract your abdominal muscles, drawing ribs and hips together.
3. Use your abs to rotate legs to the left, lifting up onto your left hip as you lift your torso up off the floor, rotating in the opposite direction (to the right); keep your abs as compressed as possible.
4. In the lifted position, you're balanced on your hips, with your entire back off the floor.
5. Hold the lifted position for a count of one-one-thousand.
6. Return to start position and alternate sides. Return to the start position after each rep.

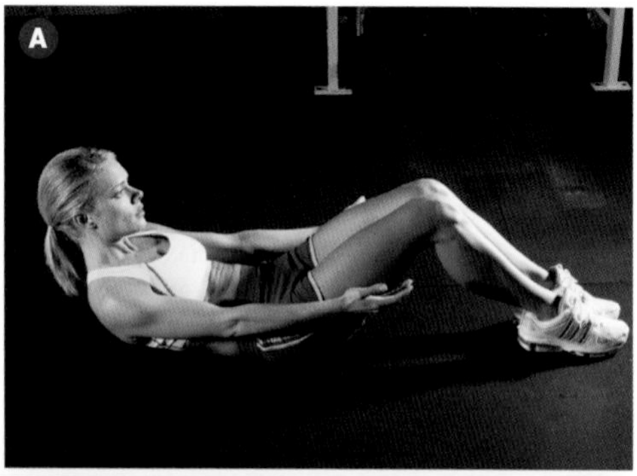


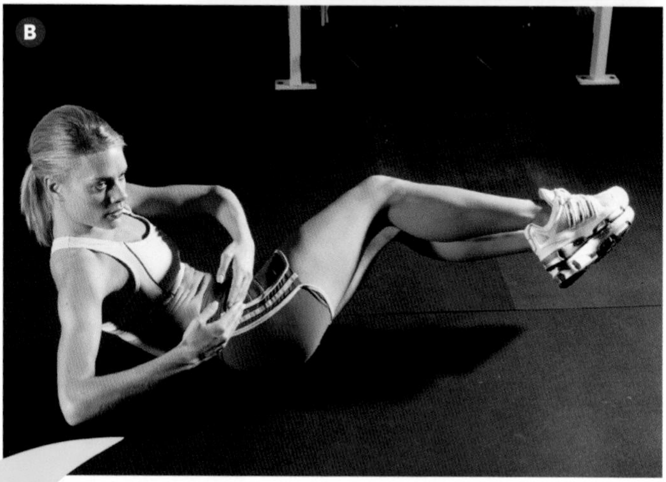


## Trainer's tips

- Keep thighs, knees and ankles squeezed together throughout the movement.
- Do not use momentum to rotate, which can cause you to lose balance or rock your hips from side to side; this prevents your abs from working maximally.
- Use slow, controlled movements rather than twisting from side to side.
- Keep your spine slightly rounded rather than perfectly straight, which can strain back muscles and ligaments.
- Think of rotating around a pivotal point, shoulders moving toward opposite hip as legs rotate in opposition.
- Beginners should keep their knees bent. For more of a challenge, lessen the knee bend so your legs are almost straight as you rotate.

### Inside Edge

***This exercise requires some balance, so coordinate the upper torso lift and rotation to occur simultaneously with the rotation of your legs.***

# Weighted Ball Crunch

BEGINNER/ INTERMEDIATE/ADVANCED

***Muscles Worked:*** *rectus abdominis, bilateral contraction of external and internal obliques, transverse abdominis*

## Technique

1. Sit upright on a stability ball, holding a dumbbell vertically on your chest with both hands. Walk feet out in front of you, letting the ball roll up your spine until torso is parallel to the floor and supported from shoulder blades to hips by ball, head and shoulders off the ball.
2. Feet are flat on floor, knees bent at 90 degrees and aligned over ankles.
3. Contract your abdominal muscles, bringing spine to a neutral position. Tuck chin in slightly, focusing on a spot straight ahead.
4. Curl torso upward, moving as one unit, only flexing from the spine.
5. Pause then lower to start position.

## Trainer's tips

- Adding weight to a basic crunch overloads your abdominal muscles with fewer reps, making this exercise more effective and time-efficient.
- When using weights, don't lower your torso too far below parallel.
- Keep head and neck aligned, shoulders drawn down from your ears, knees and feet in the same position throughout the recommended reps.
- Don't use momentum to lift your torso up against the weight; this "rock-and-roll" motion will cause the ball to roll underneath you, decreasing the exercise's effectiveness.
- To make this exercise more challenging and require more stabilization, do it with legs extended and balanced on your heels.

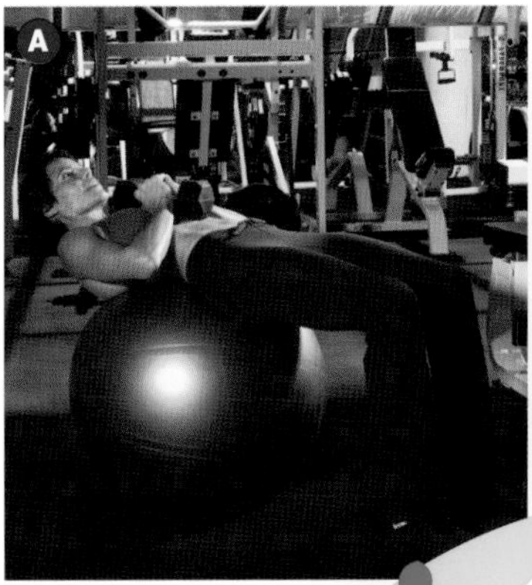


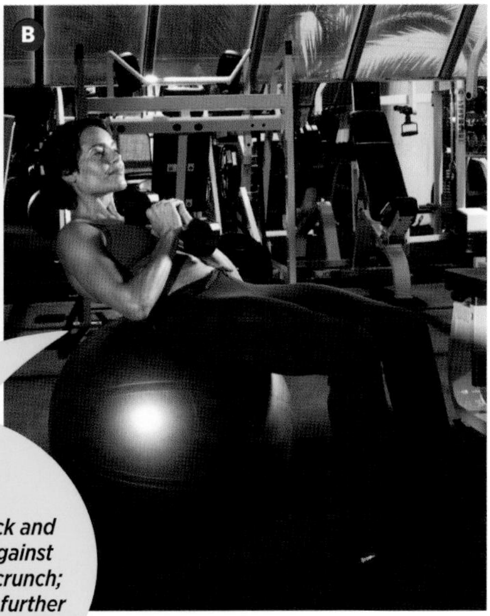


**Inside Edge**

***Keep lower back and hips pressed against the ball as you crunch; this extra effort further engages your abs.***

# Beginner Workouts

***Directions:** This is a progressive, six-week program. Do the following exercises three times per week for the first four weeks, then increase to a four-day schedule for weeks 5 and 6.*

| WEEK | EXERCISE | SETS | REPS |
|---|---|---|---|
| 1 | Half Rollback on Ball | 2 | 8–12 |
| | Cross-Body Crunch | 1–2 | 8–12 |
| 2 | Ball Crunch | 2 | 12–15 |
| | Reverse Trunk Twist | 1–2 | 12–15 |
| 3 & 4 | Weighted Ball Crunch | 2 | 10–12 |
| | Leg and Arm Press | 2 | 8–10 |
| | Plus any 2 of the 4 exercises listed for weeks 1 and 2; alternate variations each session | 2 | 10–15 |
| 5 & 6 | 4-day rotation: Do one workout each day. Perform each workout as a tri-set or circuit. (One set of each exercise with no rest between exercises equals 1 circuit.) Repeat 2–3 times, resting between circuits as needed. | | |
| | ***Workout 1*** | | **REPS** |
| | Half Rollback on Ball | | 10–15 |
| | Weighted Ball Crunch | | 8–12 |
| | Reverse Trunk Twist | | 10–15 |
| | ***Workout 2*** | | |
| | Ball Crunch | | 10–15 |
| | Cross-Body Crunch | | 10–15 |
| | Leg and Arm Press | | 10–12 |
| | ***Workout 3*** | | |
| | Cross-Body Crunch | | 10–15 |
| | Reverse Trunk Twist | | 10–15 |
| | Weighted Ball Crunch | | 8–12 |
| | ***Workout 4*** | | |
| | Leg and Arm Press | | 10–12 |
| | Half Rollback on Ball | | 12–15 |
| | Ball Crunch | | 10–15 |

**Notes**

*Rest 45–60 seconds between sets and circuits. At the end of six weeks, progress to the intermediate workouts if you're ready.*

# Intermediate Workouts

***Directions:** This is a progressive, six-week program. Do the following exercises three times per week.*

| WEEK | EXERCISE | SETS | REPS |
|---|---|---|---|
| 1 & 2 | ***Workout 1*** | | |
| | Weighted Ball Crunch | 2–3 | 10–15 |
| | Plank-to-Knee Tuck | 2 | 10–15 |
| | ***Tri-set:*** | 2 | |
| | Sidewinder | 10 | |
| | Leg and Arm Press | 10 | |
| | Scissor Cycle | 20 | |
| | Medicine-Ball Reverse Crunch | 2–3 | 10–12 |
| 3 & 4 | ***Workout 2*** | | |
| | Weighted Ball Crunch | 2–3 | 10–15 |
| | High-Cable Chop | 2–3 | 10–12 |
| | ***Compound set:*** | 2 | |
| | Medicine-Ball Oblique Crunch | 10–12 | |
| | Medicine-Ball Reverse Crunch | 10–12 | |
| | Hip Thrust | 2 | 10–12 |
| 5 & 6 | Do Workout 2 on two alternating days and Workout 1 in-between. Add a fourth day if you choose, or perform one of the Beginner Workouts for an easier abs day. | | |

***Notes***

*Rest 45–60 seconds between all sets, supersets or tri-sets. At the end of six weeks, progress to advanced workouts for more of a challenge.*

# Advanced Workouts

***Directions:** Perform two workouts a week, choosing from the following programs.*

| EXERCISE | SETS | REPS |
|---|---|---|
| ***Workout 1*** | | |
| Weighted Ball Crunch | 2-3 | 10-15 |
| Decline Weighted Twist | 2-3 | 10-15 |
| Medicine-Ball Reverse Crunch | 2-3 | 10-15 |
| Hanging Leg Raise | 2-3 | 10-15 |
| Scissor Cycle | 2-3 | 10-15 |
| ***Workout 2*** | | |
| Hanging Leg Raise | 2-3 | 10-12 |
| Plank-to-Knee Tuck | 2-3 | 10-12 |
| Medicine-Ball Reverse Crunch | 2-3 | 10-12 |
| Plank-to-Knee Tuck | 2-3 | 10-12 |
| Medicine-Ball Oblique Crunch | 2-3 | 10-12 |
| Hip Thrust | 2-3 | 10-12 |
| ***Workout 3*** | | |
| Decline Weighted Twist | 2-3 | 10-15 |
| Ball Pike | 2-3 | 10-12 |
| Weighted Ball Crunch | 2-3 | 10-15 |
| Scissor Cycle | 2-3 | 10-15 |
| Medicine-Ball Oblique Crunch | 2-3 | 10-12 |

**Notes**

*Rest 60 seconds between sets and giant sets. You can do any of these programs as straight sets or as giant sets for variety.*

# Can't-Get-to-the-Gym Workouts

***Directions:*** *Do the following exercises when you want to work out at home or on the road.*

| EXERCISE | SETS | REPS |
|---|---|---|
| ***Do the following exercises as a giant set, then repeat 2–3 times.*** | | |
| Leg and Arm Press* | | 10–12 |
| Cross-Body Crunch* | | 10–12 |
| Sidewinder | | 10–12 |
| Scissor Cycle | | 10–12 |
| Reverse Trunk Twist* | | 10–12 |
| Hip Thrust | | 10–12 |
| ***If you have a stability ball, finish with the following:*** | | |
| Ball Crunch* or Weighted Ball Crunch* | 2 | 12–15 |
| Plank-to-Knee Tuck or Ball Pike | 2 | 8–12 |

**Notes**

*Rest 60 seconds between sets and giant sets. If you're a beginner, only do the exercises marked with an asterisk (*).*

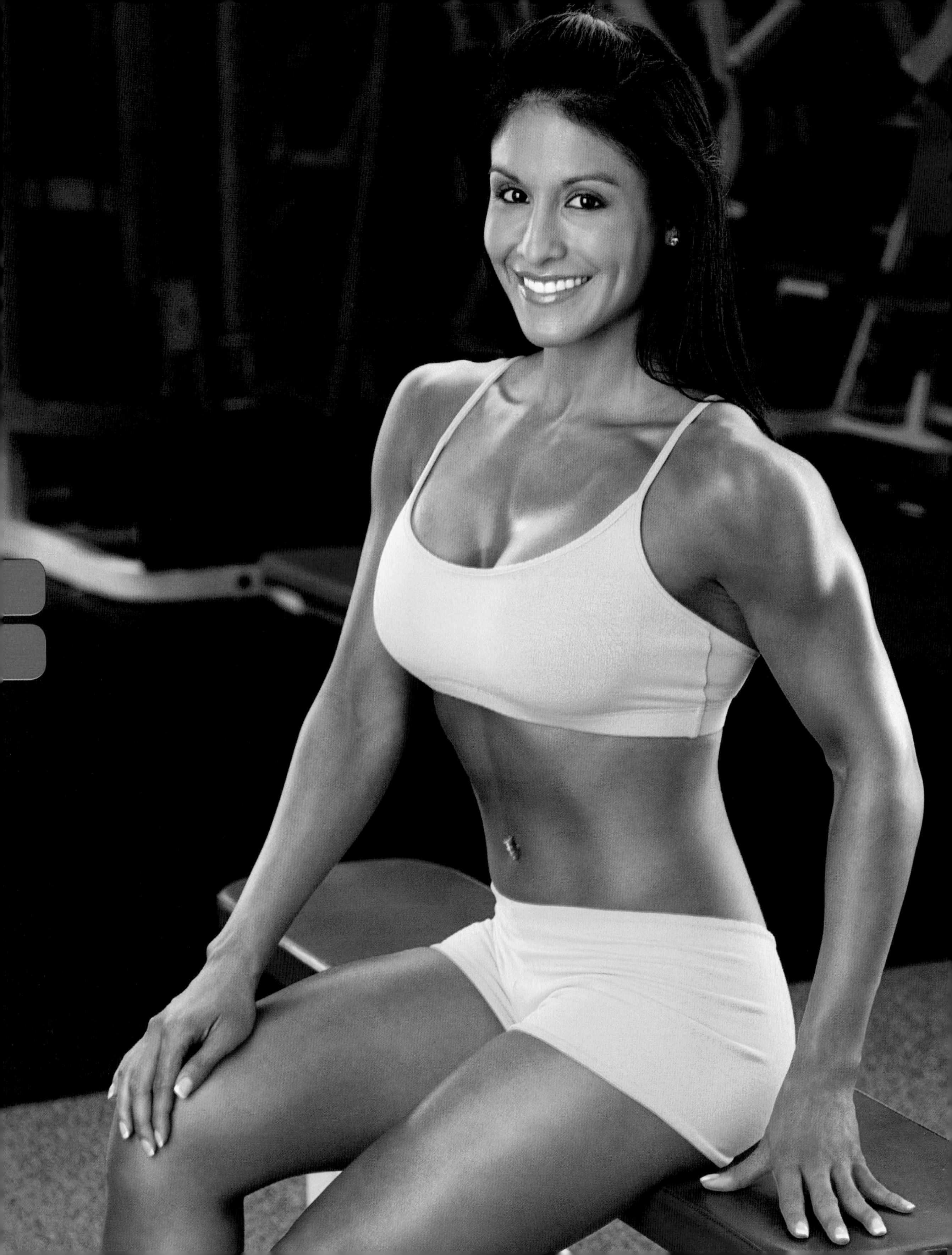

Chapter 4

# Arms

*Use essential moves to get definition in your bi's and tri's.*

THE BICEPS BRACHII AND BRACHIALIS — the muscles on the front of your upper arm — flex the elbow and rotate the forearm so your palms can face upward or downward. The biceps has a long head and a short head. Both heads cross the shoulder joint at different places, attach on the shoulder blade and insert together just below your elbow joint on the forearm. The brachialis lies under the biceps and only crosses your elbow joint. The brachioradialis, located on the thumb side of the forearm, flexes the elbow in neutral position. The triceps muscle makes up the rear of your upper arm. It is one muscle composed of three sections, joined together in one common tendon below the elbow. Together, the lateral, medial and long heads extend your elbow to straighten your arm. Both the lateral and medial heads originate on the upper arm bone (humerus), and the long head crosses the shoulder joint, attaching on the shoulder blade.

## General Guidelines for *TRAINING ARMS*

For both triceps and biceps work, keep shoulders and elbows motionless to maximize arm muscle recruitment.

Keep these muscles stimulated by regularly changing exercises, as well as equipment. For example, to work the biceps, substitute a hammer curl for a dumbbell curl or incline curl, or use cables instead of a bar.

Try doing higher reps using lighter weight every few training sessions, or, if you're trying to increase weight, use a drop set or pyramid technique.

Supersetting tri's and bi's is a highly efficient way to optimize your training, especially if you're pressed for time.

If you're at an intermediate to advanced level, try training biceps after back, or train chest with triceps on a separate day. Add an extra exercise, like a concentration curl for biceps, so you're performing three exercises, .

# Alternating Dumbbell Curl

BEGINNER/INTERMEDIATE

***Muscles Worked:*** *biceps, brachialis*

## Technique

1. Holding a dumbbell in each hand, arms extended by your sides, palms facing thighs, stand with feet hip-width apart, legs straight but not locked.
2. Contract abdominal muscles so that your spine is in a neutral position, and squeeze shoulder blades together and down to stabilize upper back.
3. Contract left biceps to bend elbow and bring dumbbell up and in toward shoulder. Rotate palm up at the top of the movement without letting torso move or elbow shift forward; keep elbow aligned with right shoulder.
4. Hold for two counts, then slowly lower and repeat, alternating sides for the set. One curl on each side equals one rep.

## Trainer's tips

- Keep shoulders square to maintain maximum workload on biceps. Shifting shoulders forward as you raise dumbbells decreases the work of the biceps and misaligns the back.
- Keep elbows aligned with shoulders and close to torso.
- Imagine a long pin going through both elbows and only allowing movement to come from the lower arm.
- For variety, do this exercise standing and using handled tubing and widen the distance between feet.
- For more of a challenge, perform standing on one foot, then standing on a balance tool such as a fitdisk or wobble board.

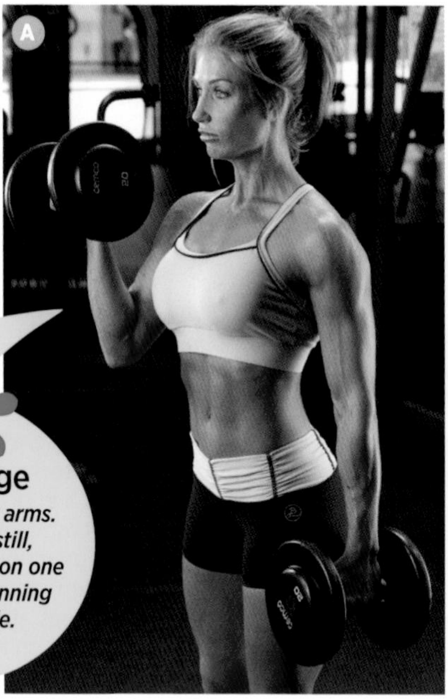


**Inside Edge**

***Don't swing your arms. To keep torso still, complete the rep on one side before beginning the other side.***

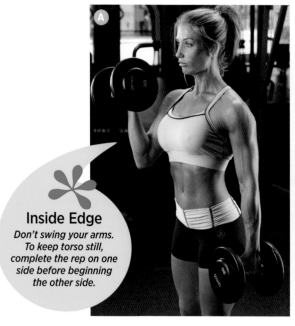

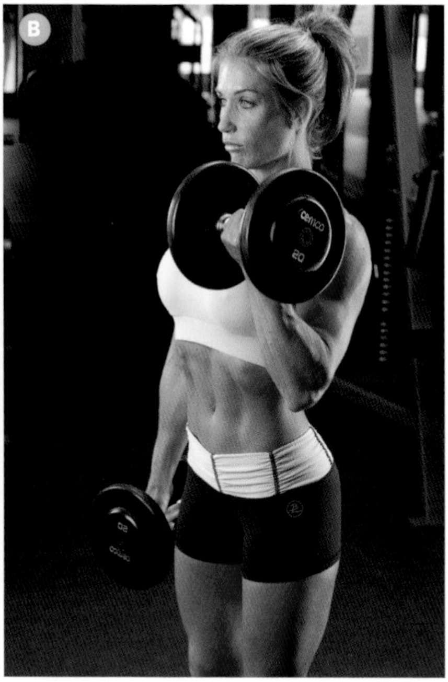

# Barbell Curl INTERMEDIATE/ADVANCED

***Muscles Worked:*** *biceps, brachialis*

## Technique

1. Stand with feet hip-width apart, knees slightly bent. Hold a barbell with an underhand grip, hands slightly wider than shoulders in a natural carrying angle, arms slightly bent.
2. Contract abdominal muscles so spine is in a neutral position, and squeeze shoulder blades down and together to stabilize upper back.
3. Align elbows under shoulders, wrists straight, chest lifted without jutting ribs out.
4. Bend elbows to bring bar up and in toward shoulders, without letting elbows drift forward or changing shoulder position. Maintain a neutral wrist position from start to finish.
5. Hold for two counts, then straighten arms to start position.

## Trainer's tips

- Keep bar level, lifting equally with both hands.
- Starting with elbows fully extended puts stress on the soft tissue of the elbow. By not locking out, you can get the benefits of a full range of motion without risking injury.
- Keeping your shoulder blades pulled back places your biceps in the best biomechanical alignment of elbows under shoulders and stabilizes your upper back, allowing you to safely handle more weight.
- Contract biceps before you lift; this ensures you're isolating your biceps without help from stronger muscles.
- When biceps fatigue, it's easy to rely on other muscles to help lift the weight. When your form falters, stop.

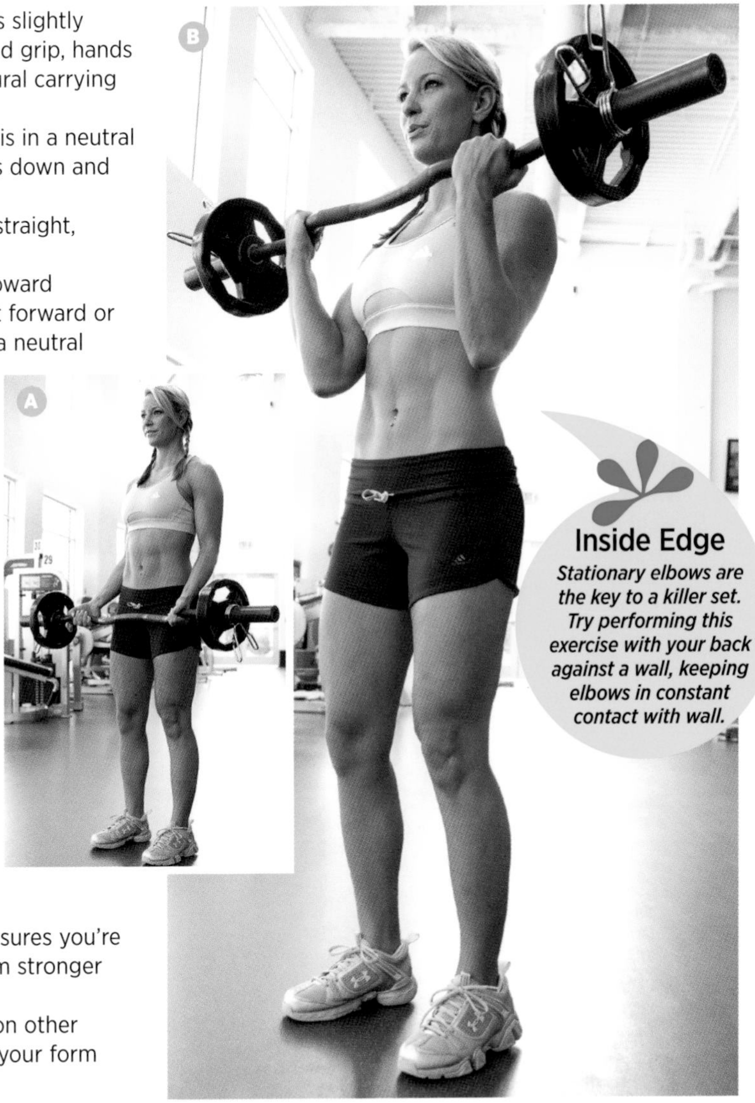


**Inside Edge**

*Stationary elbows are the key to a killer set. Try performing this exercise with your back against a wall, keeping elbows in constant contact with wall.*

# Basic Biceps Dumbbell Curl

BEGINNER/INTERMEDIATE

***Muscles Worked:** biceps, brachialis*

## Technique

1. Holding a dumbbell in each hand, stand with your feet hip-width apart, knees slightly bent and toes pointing forward.
2. Let arms hang down by your sides in a natural carrying angle, elbows aligned with shoulders and palms facing forward so thumbs point out, wrists straight.
3. Contract abdominal muscles, bringing spine to a neutral position; squeeze shoulder blades together and down to stabilize your upper back and prevent rocking.
4. Maintaining shoulder and elbow position, keep your upper arms vertical and bend your elbows, bringing dumbbells up toward your shoulders while keeping wrists straight.
5. Hold for two counts, then slowly lower to start position.

## Trainer's tips

- If your elbows drift forward, you've lost shoulder stability, allowing other muscles to assist with the movement and lessening the work of the biceps.
- Keep your body erect so your torso doesn't lean forward and back; this causes you to lose stability in your core muscles and can impede your ability to safely handle heavier weights.
- Prevent momentum from easing the biceps workload by taking longer to complete the lifting and lowering phase of each rep.
- For variety, substitute an EZ-bar, barbell, tubing or any cable attachment for dumbbells. A cable rope is especially effective.

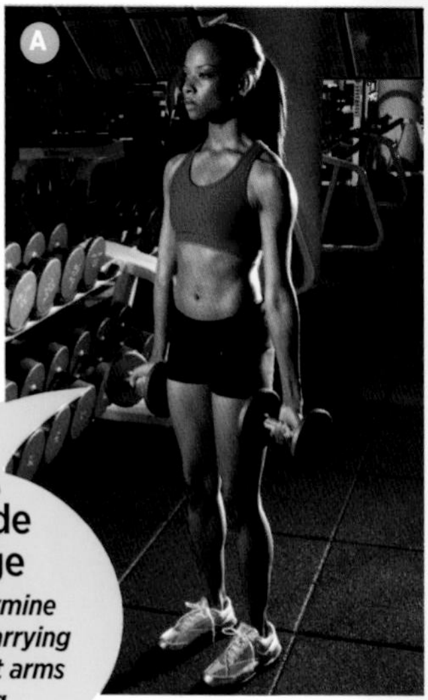


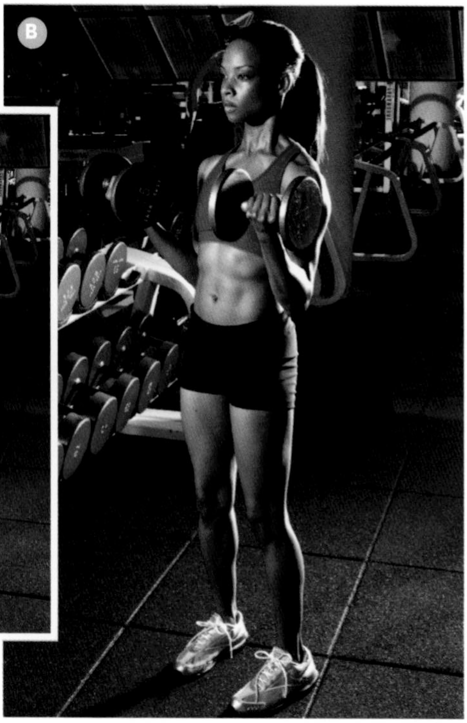


**Inside Edge**

*To determine natural carrying angle, let arms hang.*

# Bench Dip

BEGINNER/INTERMEDIATE/ADVANCED

***Muscles Worked:*** *triceps, with emphasis on lateral and medial heads*

## Technique

1. Sitting on the long edge of a flat bench with feet hip-width apart and knees extended, place hands on bench edge near hips with fingers facing forward.
2. Contract abdominal muscles so spine is neutral; squeeze shoulder blades together and down.
3. Straighten arms and lift hips, sliding forward until they are just off the edge of the bench.
4. Keeping shoulders down, bend elbows, lowering hips toward the floor without letting them drift forward, until bend in elbows approaches about 90 degrees.
5. Without using added inertia from your legs, straighten arms fully but don't lock elbows. Hold for two counts, then repeat.

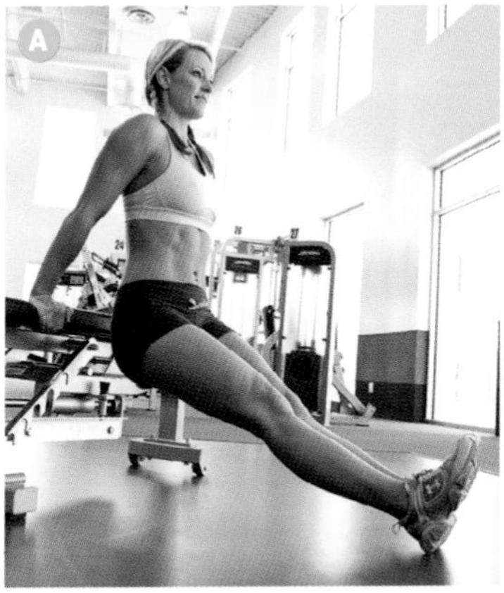


## Trainer's tips

- Keep hips as uninvolved as possible by eliminating any contribution by the quads or glutes; they'll automatically try to assist the lift if you let them.
- Keep elbows from flaring by pressing them toward each other while bending to lower position.
- If you're a beginner, keep knees in line with ankles. To increase difficulty, progressively move feet out until legs are straight, lift one foot off floor or place both feet on another bench or on a stability ball in front of you.
- For a greater challenge, perform with one or both feet on a fitdisk.
- Add weighted resistance by placing a dumbbell, plate or medicine ball across hips.

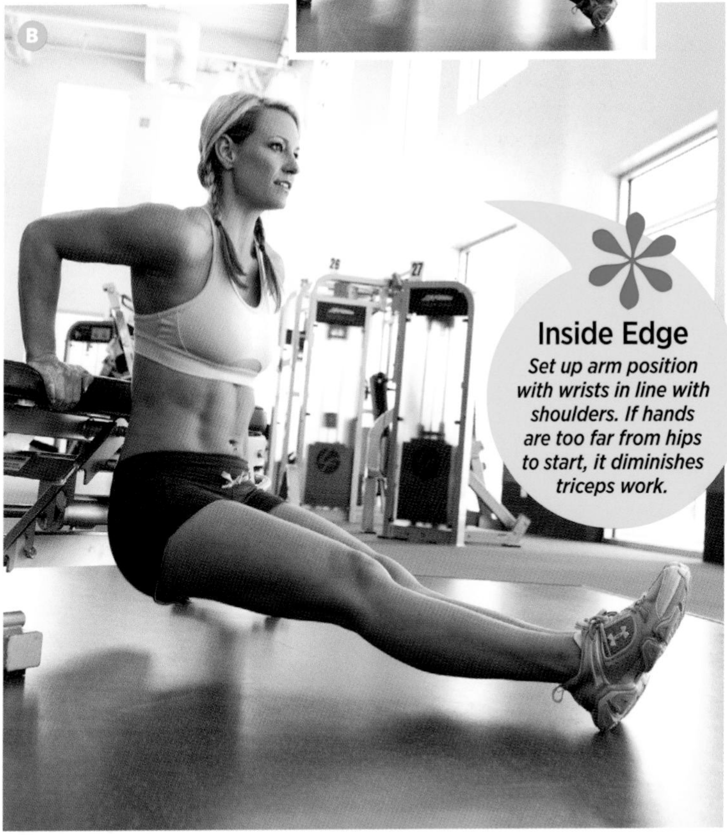


**Inside Edge**

***Set up arm position with wrists in line with shoulders. If hands are too far from hips to start, it diminishes triceps work.***

# Biceps Cable Curl INTERMEDIATE/ADVANCED

***Muscles Worked:** biceps, brachialis*

## Technique

1. Attach a straight or cambered bar to a low-cable pulley and grasp bar with both hands using an underhand grip, elbows slightly bent, wrists neutral.
2. Stand close enough to weight stack to hold elbows close to torso and in line with shoulders. Feet are separated hip-width apart, knees slightly bent.
3. Contract abdominal muscles so your spine is in a neutral position, and squeeze your shoulder blades together and down.
4. Maintain elbow, shoulder and wrist position and contract biceps to bend elbows, bringing bar up and in toward shoulders without shifting weight or leaning torso back.
5. Hold for two counts, then straighten arms to start position, resisting the forward pull of the cable.

## Trainer's tips

- You'll be less likely to lean your torso backwards if you perform this exercise with a slight bend in the knees.
- If you have wider shoulders, it may be easier to keep shoulder blades pulled back if you use the outside angled portion of the bar. Using the inner angled portion may cause your shoulders to roll forward and your elbows to flare.
- Keep elbow aligned with shoulder and make sure your working arm is lined up directly with the cable.
- For variety, try substituting a straight bar or the rope. You can also perform this exercise while sitting on a stability ball.

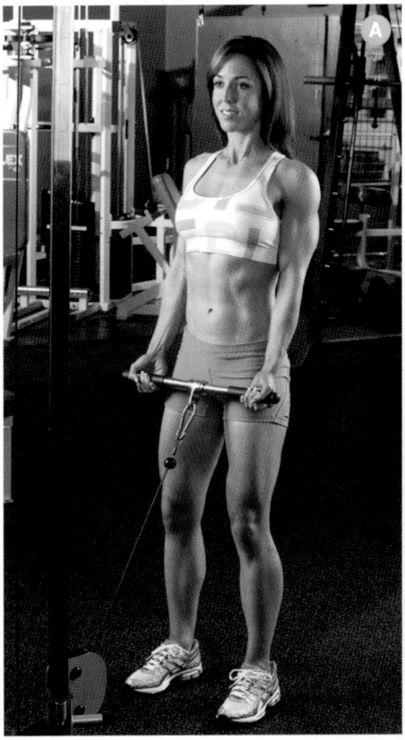


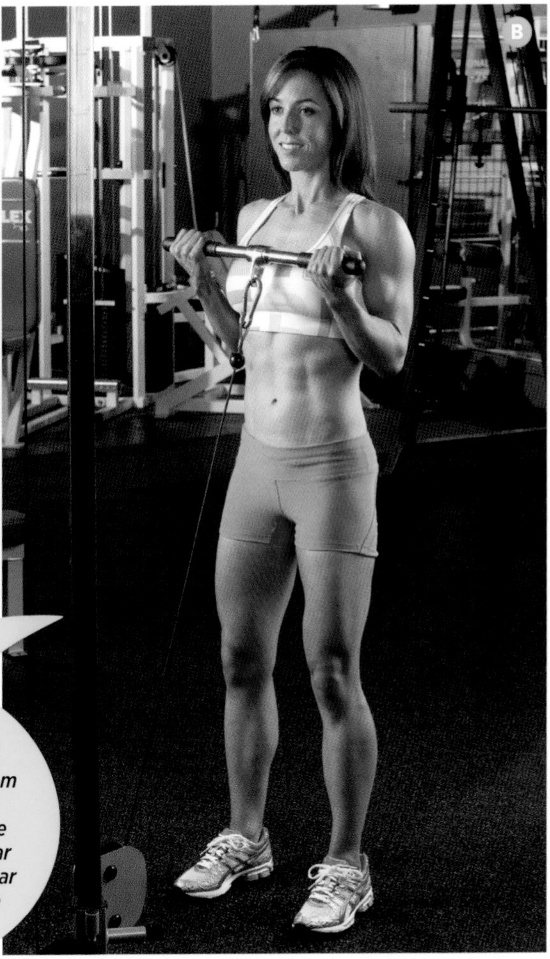


**Inside Edge**

*Standing too far from the weight stack makes this exercise easier; stand just far enough away to clear the stack with the handle.*

# Concentration Curl

BEGINNER/ INTERMEDIATE/ADVANCED

***Muscles Worked:*** *biceps, brachialis*

## Technique

1. Grasp a dumbbell with your right hand and sit on a bench, knees bent and aligned over ankles, feet slightly wider than hip-width apart.
2. Contract abdominal muscles so your spine is neutral and squeeze shoulder blades together and down to stabilize upper back.
3. With chest lifted, hinge forward from hips, keeping back flat, and place back of right upper arm against inside of right thigh. Arm hangs vertically, aligned under shoulder, wrist straight.
4. Bend elbow, bringing dumbbell up and in toward shoulder, taking care not to change shoulder of upper arm position; keep wrist neutral.
5. Hold for two counts, then slowly lower to start position. Repeat for reps, then switch arms.

## Trainer's tips

- Don't cock your wrist to increase the curl; this won't increase the exercise's effectiveness.
- Don't hyperextend your neck out of neutral position and place stress on your cervical spine. You should feel stretched in your neck while elongating the spine.
- Keep your body still as you lift and lower the dumbbell. The less extraneous body movement, the more stable you'll be, and the more weight you'll be able to lift.
- If you're advanced, you can perform this using a single handle and low cable while sitting on a stability ball. Superset with double biceps cable curl and high-pulley curl for a quick tri-set.

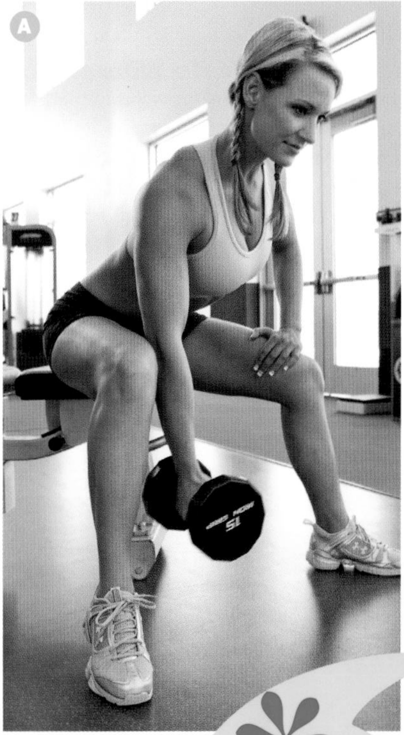


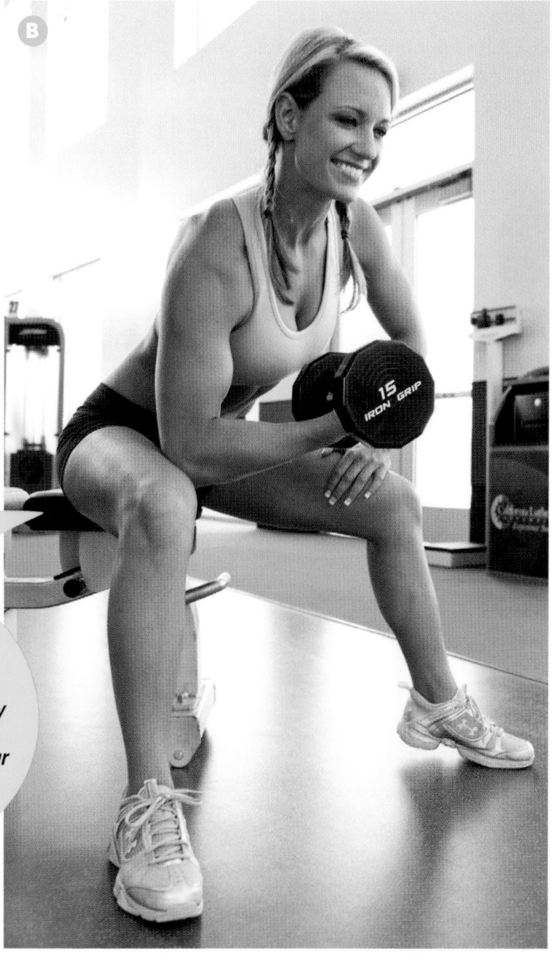


**Inside Edge**

*Retain upper arm and elbow position by firmly pressing against your thigh; this stabilizes your position so you don't "cheat."*

# Hammer Curl BEGINNER/INTERMEDIATE

***Muscles Worked:*** *biceps, with emphasis on brachialis*

## Technique

1. Holding a dumbbell in each hand, arms hanging by your sides with palms facing in, stand with feet hip-width apart, legs straight but not locked and feet pointing straight ahead.
2. Contract abdominal muscles so your spine is in neutral and squeeze shoulder blades down and together, aligning elbows and wrists under shoulders.
3. Contract biceps of one arm and bend elbow, bringing dumbbell up toward front of shoulder, palm still facing in, wrists neutral. Don't let your torso move or your elbow shift forward at the top of the movement. Alternate arms every other rep.
4. Hold for two counts at the top of the movement, then slowly lower to start position without locking elbows.

## Trainer's tips

- You'll maximize muscle fiber recruitment by keeping shoulder blades drawn down and in toward spine as you curl and release. This makes it harder for the elbows to swing forward and keeps muscle fibers in optimal alignment.
- Don't pump the weights; the only movement should be elbow flexion.
- Don't lean torso forward or over-arch lower back; this reduces your stability, making it harder to safely handle heavy weights.
- For variety, sit on a stability ball or stand using single low-cable handles, performing one arm at a time. You can also stand in the center of a handled tubing, grasping handles with palms facing in.

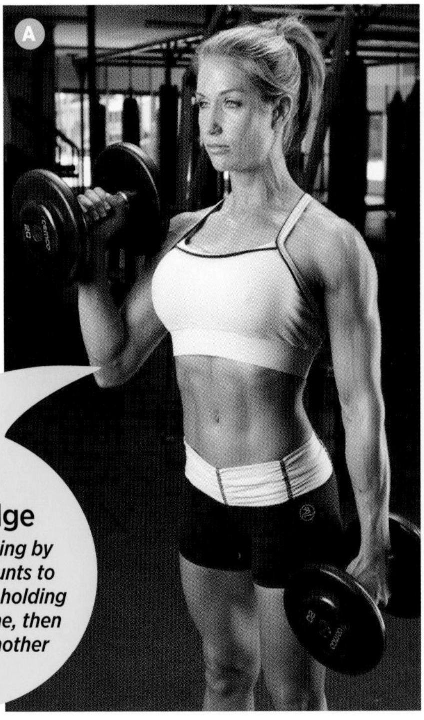


**Inside Edge**

***Minimize swinging by taking three counts to raise dumbbells, holding for a count of one, then lowering for another three.***

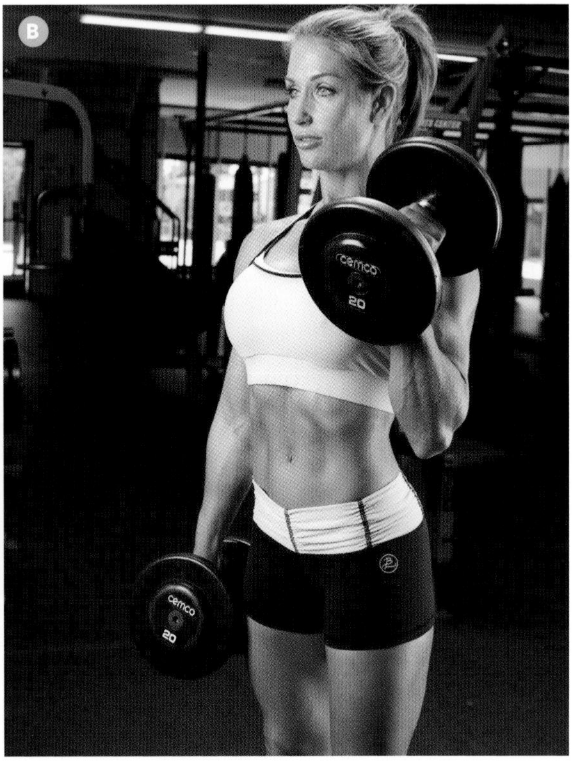

# High-Cable Curl ADVANCED

***Muscles Worked:** biceps, brachialis*

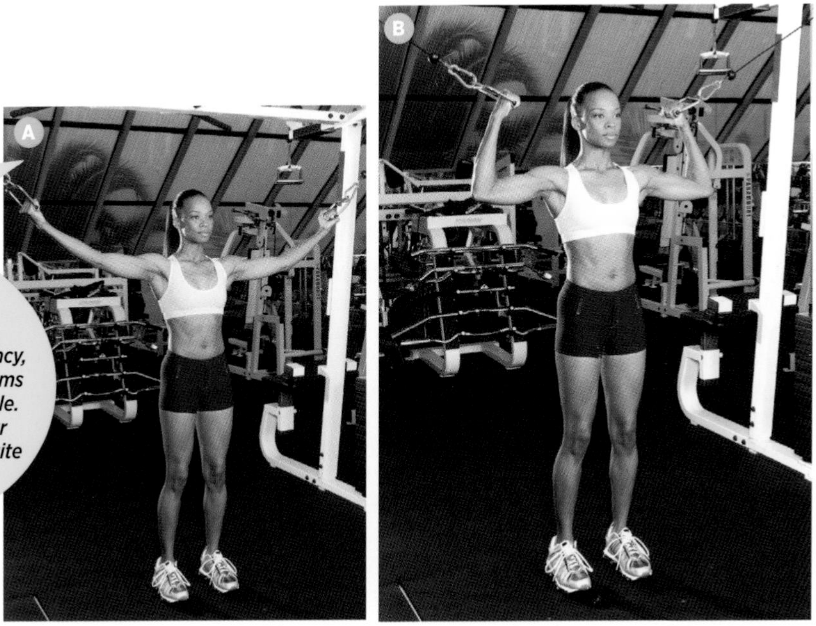


**Inside Edge**

***For maximum efficiency, line up your upper arms directly with the cable. This may mean your upper arms aren't quite horizontal.***

## Technique

1. Attach a single cable handle to each upper cable in a cable cage.
2. Grasp each handle in an underhand grip and stand centered in cage. Feet are hip-width apart, arms and shoulders aligned with cable between both weight stacks when arms are extended, wrists straight.
3. Bend elbows slightly, enough to take any strain off elbow and shoulder joints, and contract abdominals so spine is neutral; squeeze shoulder blades down and together, chest lifted and shoulders relaxed.
4. Maintaining arm position at shoulder height, bring handles toward shoulders without curling wrists or lifting elbows.
5. Pause, then slowly straighten arms to start position.

## Trainer's tips

- At the completion of the move, the two middle knuckles will face down into the top of the shoulder.
- Make sure your shoulders don't round forward as you perform this curl; this lessens the effectiveness of the biceps work and places tension on the shoulder joint.
- Avoid leaning your torso forward or back, or rocking as you curl. A staggered stance might make it easier to stabilize your torso.
- Keep your upper arms still; dropping your elbows as you perform the curl will involve the lats, and the biceps will have less work to do.
- To increase the difficulty, try the high-pulley curl using one arm at a time.

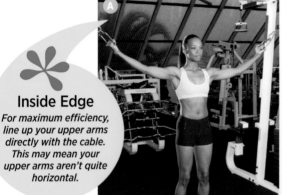

# Incline Alternating Dumbbell Curl ADVANCED

***Muscles Worked:** biceps, with emphasis on long head; brachialis*

## Technique

1. Grasping a dumbbell in each hand, sit back on an incline bench with the back adjusted so your arms hang vertically when seated without placing stress on the front of the shoulder joint (approximately 60 degrees). Knees are bent and feet are flat on floor.
2. Contract abdominal muscles so spine is neutral, and squeeze shoulder blades down and together.
3. Let arms hang straight down toward the floor, aligned with shoulders, elbows slightly bent, palms facing forward, wrists neutral.
4. Bend one elbow, bringing dumbbell up and in toward shoulder without letting elbow drift forward. Wrist remains straight.
5. Pause, slowly lower to start position, and repeat with other arm to complete one rep.

## Trainer's tips

- While a full range of motion is optimum, an extreme range of motion can cause injury. Adjust incline so you don't feel any shoulder discomfort, and the focus is entirely on the biceps.
- To help keep shoulders square, completely finish the rep on one side before beginning rep on other side.
- While straining to finish the last rep or two, tighten your abs to give you the additional stability to finish the rep.
- To increase the intensity, lift one foot slightly off floor for duration of set.

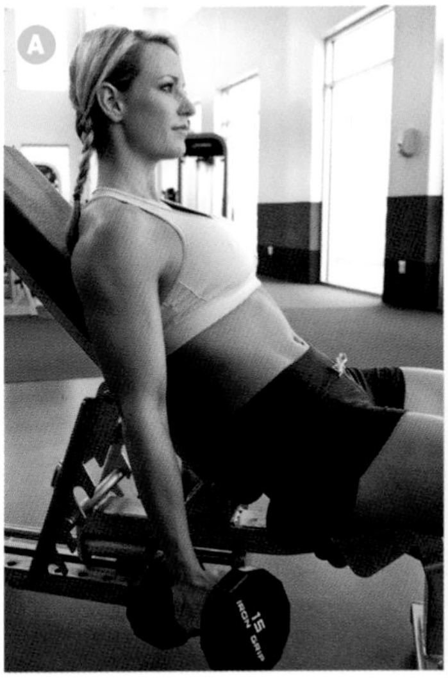


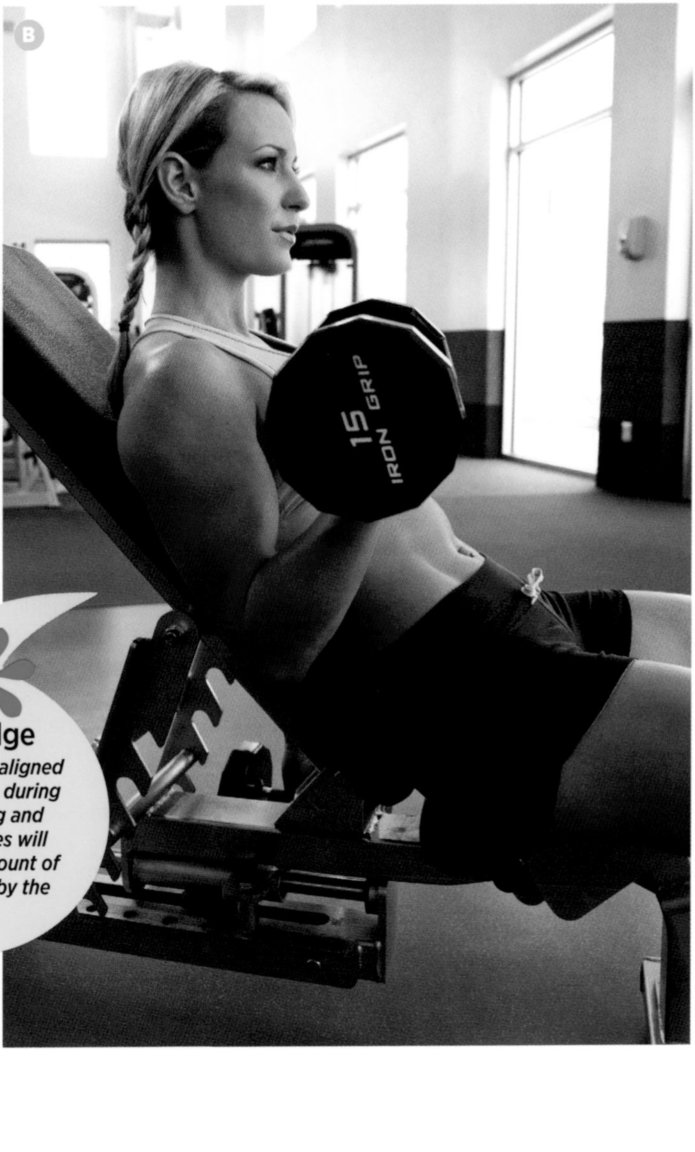


**Inside Edge**

*Keeping elbows aligned under shoulders during both the lifting and lowering phases will increase the amount of work required by the biceps.*

# Lying Overhead Dumbbell Press

BEGINNER/INTERMEDIATE

*Muscles Worked: triceps, with emphasis on long head*

## Technique

1. Lie faceup on a flat bench with your knees bent and feet on the floor or edge of the bench. Hold a dumbbell in each hand, palms facing in, arms extended straight in the air and in line with your shoulders.
2. Contract abdominal muscles so your spine is in a neutral position. Stabilize shoulder blades by bringing them down and in toward spine.
3. Bend your elbows, bringing the head of the dumbbells back and down toward shoulders in an arc without changing elbow or shoulder position, elbows pointing toward ceiling.
4. Use your triceps muscles to fully straighten arms to start position without locking your elbows.

## Trainer's tips

- To keep elbows from flaring and taking arms out of alignment, keep upper arms parallel and pressing toward each other.
- Keep abs firmly contracted and avoid lowering dumbbells too far behind you, which can cause the back to arch, taking you out of a neutral and protected spine position.
- For variety, try substituting the dumbbells with an EZ-bar, a barbell or even a medicine ball. Or, place a bench in front of a low-cable stack and perform with head facing weight stack using a bar or single handle.
- For more of a challenge, lift feet off bench or perform on a stability ball.

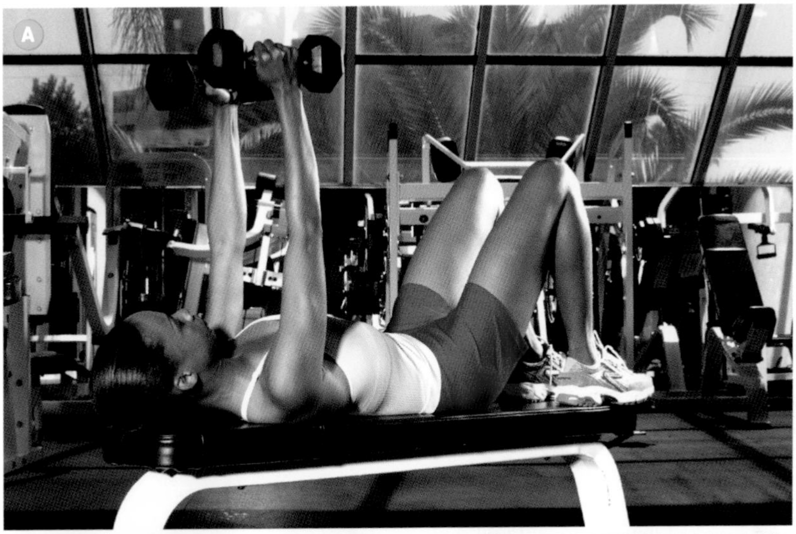


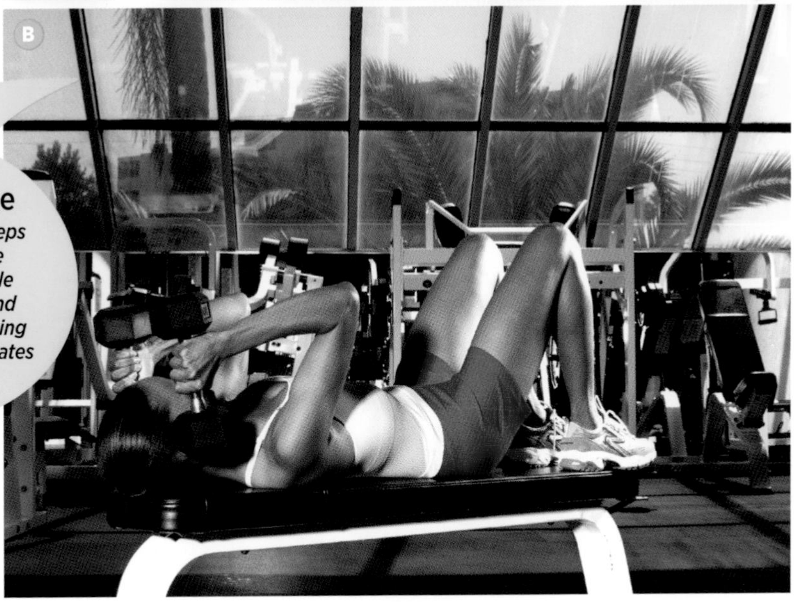


**Inside Edge**

*To maximize triceps work, keep the elbows still while straightening and bending. Stabilizing the elbows eliminates momentum.*

# Lying Triceps Extension

INTERMEDIATE/ADVANCED

***Muscles Worked:** triceps, with emphasis on long head*

## Technique

1. Grasp an EZ-bar with an overhand grip and lie faceup on a bench, knees bent and feet on edge of bench or floor. Lift bar overhead, arms straight and aligned over shoulders, wrists in a neutral position.
2. Contract abdominal muscles so spine is in a neutral position, and squeeze shoulder blades down and together.
3. While keeping elbows pressed toward each other, bend them and lower bar toward forehead without changing shoulder or elbow position. Upper arms will be vertical, elbows pointing to the ceiling.
4. Contract triceps to straighten arms and press bar back up to start position without locking elbows.
5. Hold for two counts, then lower and return to start position.

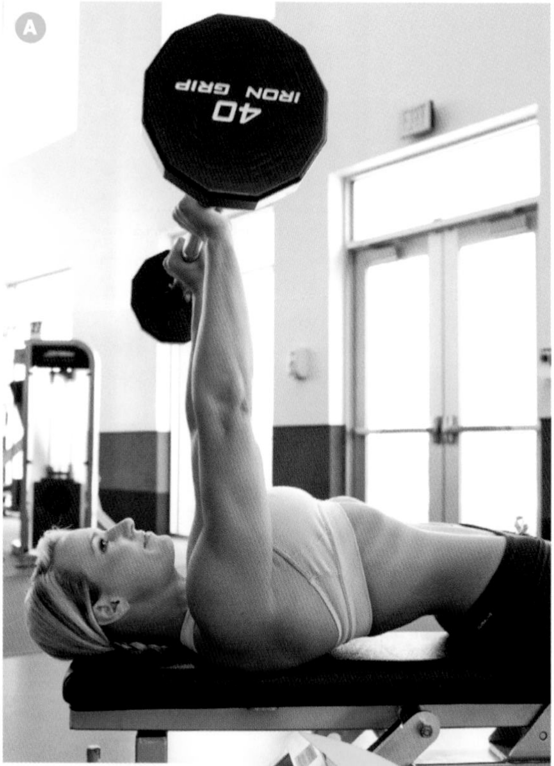


## Trainer's tips

- Don't allow back to arch as you lower bar, and don't tuck pelvis as you extend. This makes you less stable and can also strain your back.
- For variety, substitute a barbell or a large medicine ball. You can also do this exercise with a low cable. Attach the cambered bar to a low-cable pulley and lie on bench with top of your head facing the weight stack.
- For more of a challenge, lift both feet and hold lower legs parallel to floor or lie on a fitdisk or airex pad; this will force your core muscles to work harder to compensate for the decreased stability.
- To increase difficulty, substitute a stability ball for the bench.

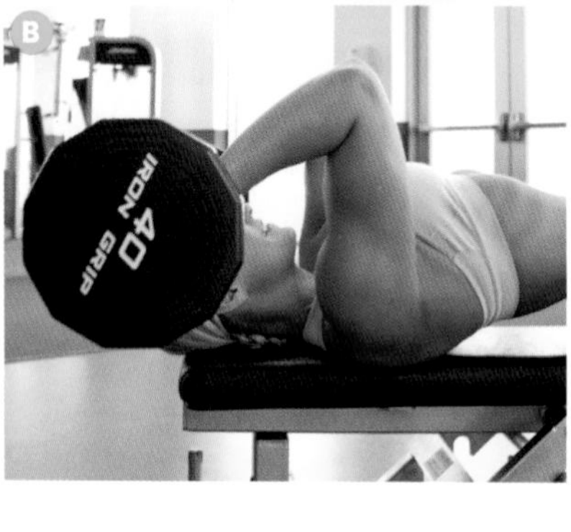


**Inside Edge**

***Maintain vertical upper-arm position to keep workload on triceps; unnecessary drifting of elbows forward or back will bring other muscles into play.***

# Prone Triceps Extension

INTERMEDIATE/ADVANCED

***Muscles Worked:*** *triceps*

## Technique

1. Lie facedown on a flat bench with your chin just over bench edge, legs extended and feet together.
2. Hold a dumbbell in each hand, palms facing in, elbows bent at 90-degree angles and close to your sides. Upper arms are parallel to the floor, knuckles pointing down.
3. Contract abdominal muscles to bring spine into neutral, dropping tailbone; roll shoulders back and down, squeezing shoulder blades together.
4. Keeping shoulders and elbows still, straighten both arms behind you without locking elbows, keeping head of dumbbells pointing toward the floor, wrists straight.
5. Hold for two counts, then bend elbows to start position.

## Trainer's tips

- Keep back of neck long with nose facing the bench to avoid placing stress on the neck.
- If you experience any lower-back discomfort, place a rolled-up towel under your pelvis, or perform the exercise lying facedown on a stability ball.
- Keeping the motion of the dumbbells slow and controlled will force the triceps to do more work. Swinging creates momentum and actually takes a portion of the workload away from the triceps.
- For variety, rotate palms up to face the ceiling by the end of the move, or start with palms facing forward.
- Superset this exercise with a prone dumbbell lat row or a prone flye.

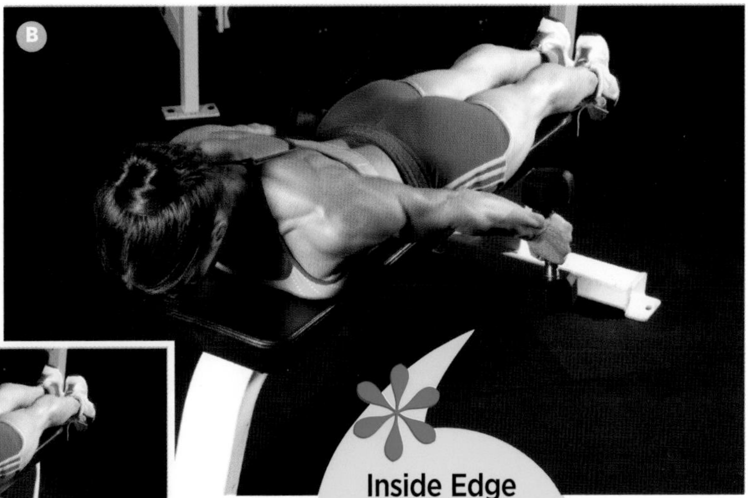


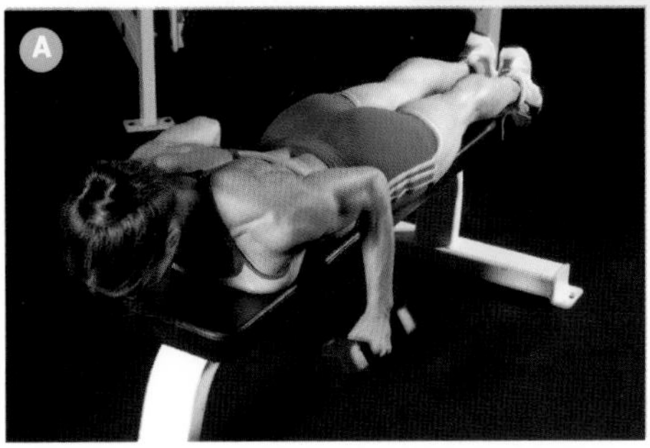


**Inside Edge**
*Use your back and shoulder muscles to stabilize upper-arm position so you can fully extend arm to parallel.*

# Rotating French Press ADVANCED

***Muscles Worked:*** *triceps, with emphasis on long head*

## Technique

1. Lie faceup on a flat bench, knees bent, feet on bench edge or floor. Hold a dumbbell in each hand, palms facing feet with arms extended straight up in the air and in line with shoulders.
2. Contract abdominal muscles so your spine is in a neutral position, and squeeze shoulder blades together and down to stabilize upper back.
3. Bend elbows, rotating lower arms so that palms face you and knuckles are just above forehead in the final position without changing elbow or shoulder position; elbows should be pointing at the ceiling.
4. Straighten arms without locking elbows, rotating palms out by the end of the movement.

## Trainer's tips

- Minimize momentum and maximize workload on the triceps by engaging the lats and shoulder muscles to stabilize the upper arm and the shoulder joint.
- For variety, try using a cabled weight stack. Attach a single handle to the low pulley. Place a flat bench lengthwise and lay with top of head next to stack.
- For more of a challenge, lift feet and keep knees bent at 90 degrees. You can also increase the difficulty by lying on a fitdisk or doing the exercise on a stability ball.
- For a killer tri-set, combine with one set of prone triceps extensions and a set of bench dips.

### Inside Edge

***The rotation of your arm occurs at the shoulder joint; keep upper arm vertical and wrists straight without snapping your elbows.***

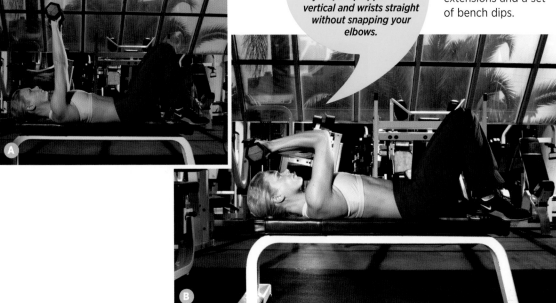

# Triceps Kickback

BEGINNER/ INTERMEDIATE/ADVANCED

***Muscles Worked:*** *triceps*

## Technique

1. Holding a dumbbell in left hand, stand at arm's distance from a low-back seat or inclined bench with back of bench adjusted to a lower position. Feet are hip-width apart.
2. Contract abdominal muscles to bring spine to neutral position. Lift chest, squeezing shoulder blades together and down.
3. Bend knees, hinging forward from hips until back is parallel to floor, placing right hand on back of bench.
4. Bend left elbow close to torso so upper arm is parallel to floor, knuckles pointing down toward floor. Straighten left arm, bringing dumbbell back and up until arm is fully extended, but not locked.
5. Hold for two counts, then slowly bend elbow to start position. Do all reps, and then switch sides.

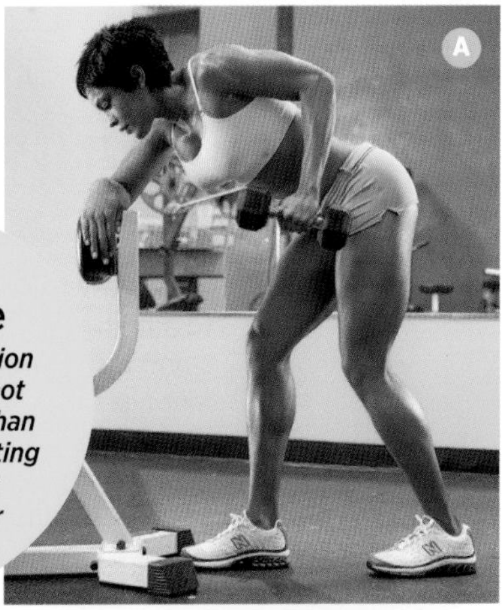


**Inside Edge**

***Keep constant tension on the triceps by not lifting arm higher than parallel position; lifting above this point engages the rear deltoid.***

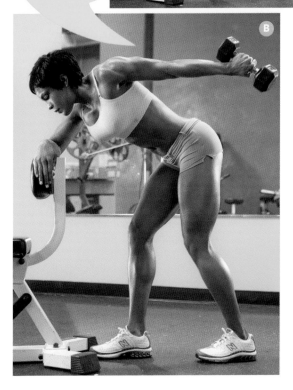


## Trainer's tips

- If you're having trouble maintaining a neutral spine and are rounding your back, you may have tight hamstrings. Try to remedy the situation by bending knees more and performing hamstring stretches.
- Don't use so much weight that you're unable to fully straighten your arm.
- For variety, do this exercise using tubing, or at the low-cable stack with a single handle attached and pulling the bench up lengthwise in front of stack.
- You can also perform this as a two-arm kickback without holding on, or rotating palms up at the end of the movement.
- For more of a challenge, substitute a stability ball for the bench.

# Triceps Pressdown

BEGINNER/ INTERMEDIATE/ADVANCED

***Muscles Worked:** triceps, with emphasis on the lateral head*

## Technique

1. Attach a V-bar or cambered bar to a high-cable pulley, then stand facing weight stack with feet hip-width apart and knees slightly bent. Contract abdominal muscles, bringing spine to a neutral position. Lift chest, squeezing shoulder blades together and down.
2. Grasping bar with an overhand grip, hands about shoulder-width apart, bend elbows, aligning them under shoulders so upper arms are close to torso in a vertical position, forearms parallel and wrists in neutral position.
3. Straighten arms, pressing bar down toward front of thighs, keeping wrists straight, palms facing thighs.
4. Hold for a count of two, then slowly bend elbows without changing shoulder or elbow alignment.

## Trainer's tips

- Minimize elbow drift by making an extra effort to stabilize your upper arms at the shoulder joint. Keep elbows still by contracting lats and rear delts and making sure shoulder blades remain squeezed together.
- Maintain an erect position; avoid leaning torso forward or over-arching back, which puts unnecessary stress on the lower back.
- For variety, do the same exercise using a straight bar or a rope; you can also do one arm at a time.
- For more of a challenge, stand with both feet on a wobble board or airex pad.
- Try this at home with handled tubing, using a door attachment between the door and the door frame.

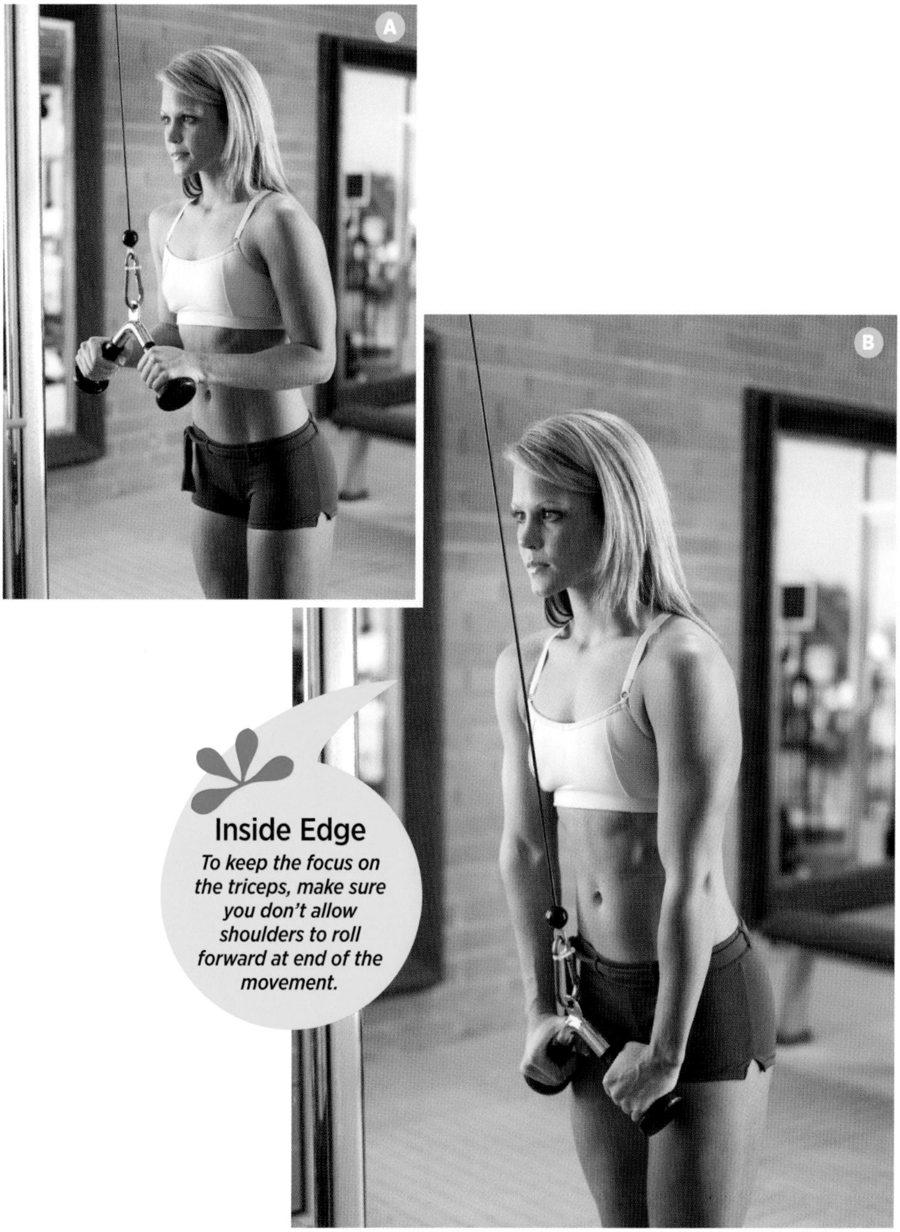


**Inside Edge**

***To keep the focus on the triceps, make sure you don't allow shoulders to roll forward at end of the movement.***

## Beginner Workouts

***Directions:* This is a progressive, six-week program. Do the following exercises twice a week. Rest 45–60 seconds between sets.**

| WEEK | EXERCISE | SETS | REPS |
|---|---|---|---|
| 1 & 2 | Triceps Pressdown | 1–2 | 10–12 |
| | Concentration Curl | 1–2 | 10–12 |
| | Lying Overhead Dumbbell Press | 1–2 | 10–12 |
| | Hammer Curl | 1–2 | 10–12 |
| 3 & 4 | Bench Dip | 1–2 | 10–15 |
| | Basic Biceps Curl | 2 | 10–15 |
| | Triceps Kickback | 2 | 10–15 |
| | Alternating Dumbbell Curl | 1–2 | 10–15 |
| 5 & 6 | ***Day 1 Workout*** | | |
| | Triceps Pressdown | 2 | 8–12 |
| | Bench Dip | 2 | 10–12 |
| | Alternate Dumbbell Curl | 2 | 10–15 |
| | Concentration Curl | 2 | 8–12 |
| | ***Day 2 Workout*** | | |
| | Basic Biceps Curl | 2 | 10–12 |
| | Hammer Curl | 2 | 10–15 |
| | Triceps Pressdown | 2 | 10–12 |
| | Triceps Kickback | 2 | 10–15 |

***Notes***

*Complement these biceps and triceps exercises with shoulder work: 1–2 sets of 10–15 reps of machine or seated dumbbell overhead presses, bent-over side lateral raises and prone flyes. At the end of six weeks, progress to intermediate workouts if you're ready.*

# Intermediate Workouts

***Directions:** This is a progressive, six-week, moderate-weight program. Do the following exercises twice per week. For lighter or heavier weights, adjust the reps accordingly.*

| WEEK | EXERCISE | SETS | REPS |
|---|---|---|---|
| 1 & 2 | Prone Triceps Extension | 2-3 | 10-12 |
| | Triceps Pressdown | 2 | 10-12 |
| | Biceps Cable Curl | 2-3 | 10-12 |
| | Bench Dip | 2 | 10-15 |
| | Concentration Curl | 2-3 | 10-12 |
| | Barbell Curl | 2 | 10-12 |
| 3 & 4 | Triceps Kickback | 2-3 | 10-15 |
| | Lying Triceps Extensions | 2-3 | 8-12 |
| | Triceps Pressdown (with rope) | 2 | 10-12 |
| | Barbell Curl | 2-3 | 8-12 |
| | Alternating Dumbbell Curl | 2-3 | 8-12 |
| | Hammer Curl | 2 | 10-12 |
| 5 & 6 | *Day 1 Workout* | | |
| | ***Superset:*** | 2-3 | |
| | Triceps Pressdown | | 8-12 |
| | Biceps Cable Curl | | 8-12 |
| | ***Superset:*** | 2 | |
| | Bench Dip | | 10-15 |
| | Lying Overhead Dumbbell Press | | 10-12 |
| | ***Superset:*** | 2 | |
| | Alternating Dumbbell Curl | | 10-12 |
| | Barbell Curl (with EZ-bar) | | 8-12 |
| | *Day 2 Workout* | | |
| | ***Superset*** | 2-3 | |
| | Lying Triceps Extension | | 8-12 |
| | Basic Biceps Dumbbell Curl | | 8-12 |
| | ***Superset*** | 2-3 | |
| | Prone Triceps Extension | | 10-12 |
| | Concentration Curl | | 8-12 |
| | Triceps Pressdown | 1st | 6-8 |
| | (decrease weight, increase reps per set) | 2nd | 8-10 |
| | | 3rd | 12-15 |
| | Biceps Cable Curl | 2 | 8-12 |

**Notes**

*Rest 45-60 seconds between sets. At the end of six weeks, progress to advanced workouts if you're ready.*

## Advanced Workouts

***Directions:* Perform two of the following workouts twice a week, using moderate weight. Work biceps and triceps on the same day, or train biceps on the same day you work back and triceps on the same day you train chest for a split. Adjust reps if you're using lighter or heavier weights.**

| EXERCISE | SETS | REPS |
|---|---|---|
| ***Workout 1*** | | |
| Triceps Pressdown | 1st | 12–15 |
| (increase weight, decrease reps per set) | 2nd | 8–10 |
| | 3rd | 6–8 |
| Bench Dip | 3 | 10–15 |
| French Press | 3 | 8–12 |
| Barbell Curl | 1st | 12–15 |
| (increase weight, decrease reps per set) | 2nd | 8–10 |
| | 3rd | 6–8 |
| Incline Alternating Dumbbell Curl | 3 | 8–12 |
| High-Cable Pulley Curl | 1st | 10–12 |
| (increase weight, decrease reps per set) | 2nd | 8–10 |
| | 3rd | 6–8 |
| ***Workout 2*** | | |
| Incline Alternating Dumbbell Curl | 3 | 10–12 |
| Biceps Cable Curl | 3 | 10–12 |
| Concentration Curl | 3 | 8–12 |
| Lying Triceps Extension | 3 | 10–12 |
| Triceps Kickback | 3 | 10–12 |
| Bench Dip | 3 | 10–12 |
| ***Workout 3*** | | |
| ***Superset:*** | 2–3 | |
| High-Cable Pulley Curl | | 10–12 |
| Biceps Cable Curl | | 10–12 |
| Barbell Curl | 3 | 8–12 |
| French Press | 3 | 8–12 |
| (or superset Barbell Curl with French Presses) | | |
| Triceps Pressdown | 3 | 10–12 |
| Prone Triceps Extension | 3 | 10–12 |

***Notes***

*Rest 45–60 seconds between sets.*

## Can't-Get-to-the-Gym Workouts

***Directions:* Do the following exercises when you want to work out at home or on the road. For variety, change the order, alternate biceps and triceps exercises, or separate them for straight sets or giant sets.**

| EXERCISE | SETS | REPS |
|---|---|---|
| Lying Overhead Dumbbell Press* or French Press | 2–3 | 10–15 |
| Triceps Kickback* | 2–3 | 10–15 |
| Bench Dip* (use a sturdy chair) | 2–3 | 10–15 |
| Basic Biceps Dumbbell Curl* or Concentration Curl | 2–3 | 10–15 |
| Hammer Curl* or Alternating Dumbbell Curl* | 2–3 | 10–15 |

**Notes**

*Rest 60 seconds between sets or giant sets. If you're a beginner, only do the exercises marked with an asterisk (*) and only choose two exercises per muscle group.*

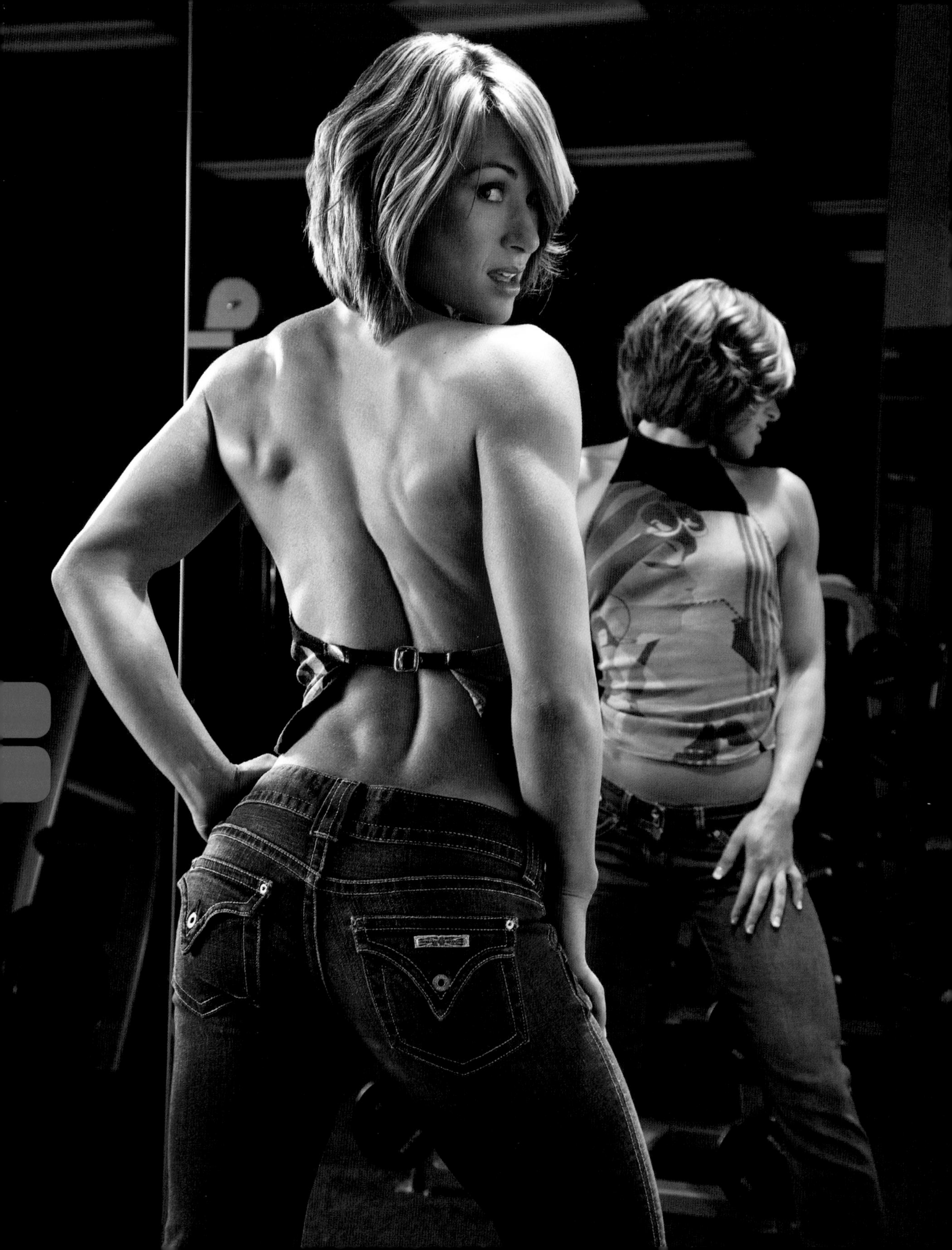

Chapter 5

# Back

*Power up your posture with a strong back.*

THE TRAPEZIUS AND RHOMBOID MUSCLES comprise your upper back. The trapezius attaches to the base of your skull, midback vertebrae and collarbone. The upper portion is involved in overhead pushing actions; the middle draws your shoulder blades back; and the lower region draws your arms back. The rhomboids lie horizontally underneath the trapezius, pulling your shoulder blades back and down.

The latissimus dorsi (lats) covers the lower and middle portions of the back. It originates on the spine, at the top of the hipbone, and attaches to the upper arm. The lats move the upper arm downward, pull the elbows down and inward, and the arms behind you, and assist the shoulders with inward rotation. Teres major, a small muscle attached on the inside of the shoulder blade, performs the same movements. The deltoids are involved with most back exercises; the lats are assisted by the biceps during any pulling actions.

The spine extensors are three muscle pairs, collectively known as the erector spinae. They run from hip to neck on either side of your spine, branching off to attach at the ribs and spine. These muscles, along with your abdominal muscles, act as stabilizers to keep the spine erect in almost all training movements.

## General Guidelines for *TRAINING BACK*

For complete back development, train two days a week, making sure to include a variety of exercises that hit all your back muscles.

If your upper-back muscles are weak or your shoulders round forward, you may want to perform more upper-back exercises than chest exercises in your routine to balance out these opposing muscle groups.

Besides altering sets, reps and weights, regularly change your back training by varying grip width (narrow, medium, wide), grip position (pronated, supinated or alternating grip), speed of movement and angle of pull.

# Angled Pulldown INTERMEDIATE/ADVANCED

***Muscles Worked:** latissimus dorsi, teres major, rear deltoid; rhomboids and middle trapezius as stabilizers; biceps assist pulling action*

## Technique

1. Attach a two-handled angled bar to a high-cable pulley. Taking a neutral grip on handles, palms facing in, sit down and position thighs under the pads. Keep feet flat on floor, knees bent and in line with ankles.
2. Lean entire torso slightly back from your hips, positioning the handles in line with your breastbone, arms straight, wrists neutral.
3. Contract your abdominal muscles, keeping chest lifted and shoulder blades drawn down and together.
4. Contract your lats, then bend elbows down and in toward waist, aligning elbows with shoulders. Pull handles down toward your collarbone as you lift chest up toward them.
5. Pause, then straighten arms to start position.

## Trainer's tips

- If your shoulders are tight, this is a great pulldown variation to include.
- Drive your elbows straight down so elbows point toward the floor in the final position; avoid pulling elbows back behind you, which can place stress on your front delts.
- Don't hunch your back or round your shoulders; these pitfalls compromise your posture and make it difficult to perform this exercise with good form.
- Keep as much space between your ears and shoulders as you can; your neck should remain long, shoulders pressed down and away from your ears.
- For variety, use a long bar attachment with both overhand and reverse grips, an angled bar, a rope or a single handle.

**Inside Edge**

***As you pull the handles toward your collarbone, press downward with your lats; continue to lift your chest upward toward the handles.***

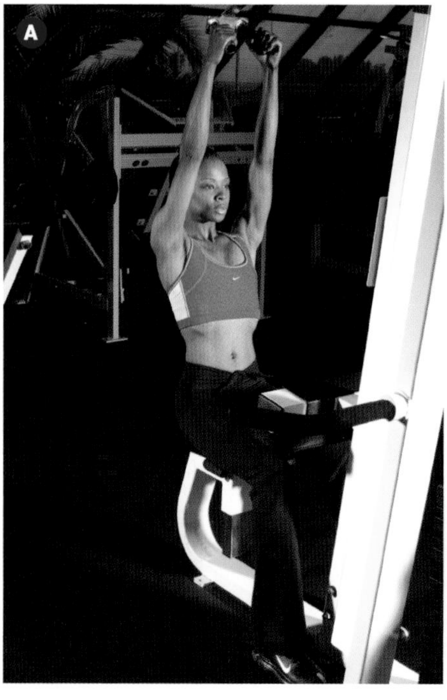


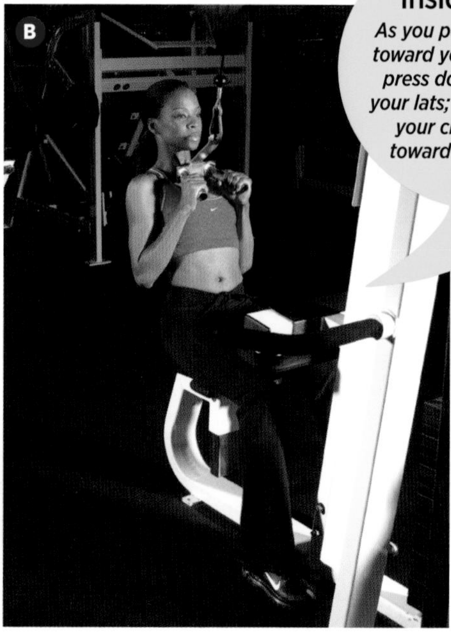

# Assisted Pull-Up BEGINNER /INTERMEDIATE

***Muscles Worked:*** *latissimus dorsi, teres major; lower fibers of trapezius; rhomboids and middle trapezius as stabilizers; biceps assist pulling action*

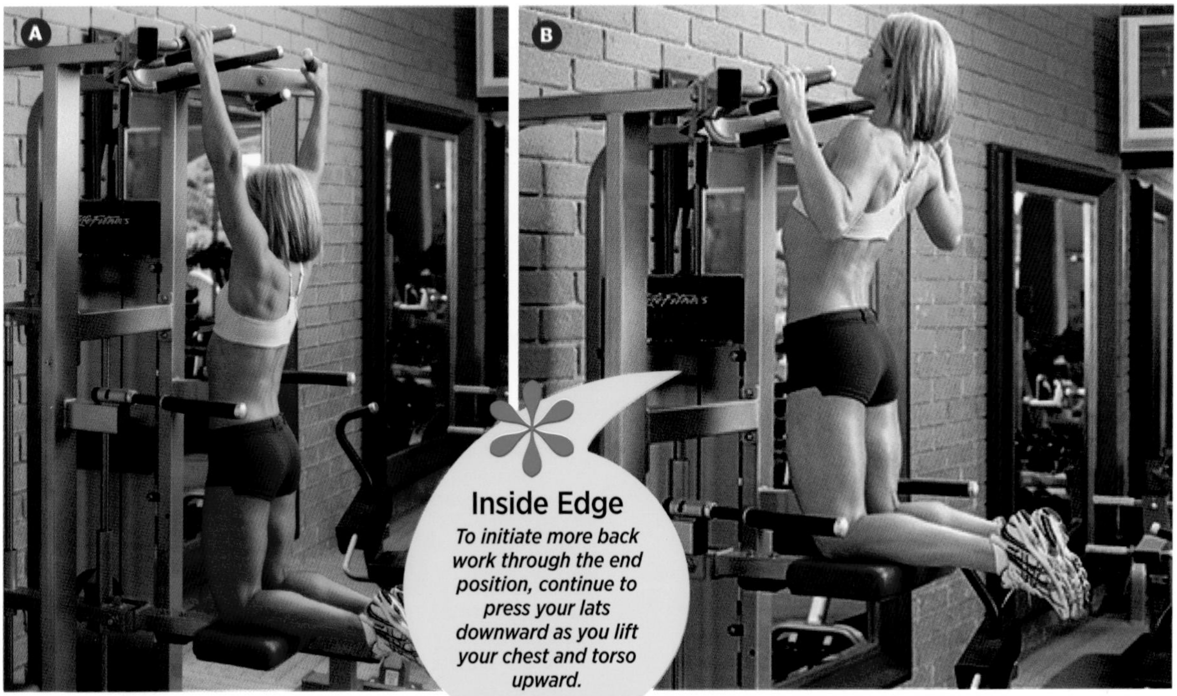


**Inside Edge**

***To initiate more back work through the end position, continue to press your lats downward as you lift your chest and torso upward.***

## Technique

1. Stand or kneel on platform (depending on machine) with feet (or knees) and hips under shoulders. Grasp overhead grips, elbows extended, palms facing in.
2. Contract abdominal muscles so spine is neutral, then lean slightly back from your ankles (if standing) or from hips (if kneeling), so hands are just in front of shoulders.
3. Pull shoulder blades down and away from ears; maintain downward squeeze for entire exercise, abs tightened to keep torso from swinging.
4. Pull yourself up, driving elbows toward your waist as you lift chest up toward the grips. Finish with elbows close to your sides, pointing down.
5. Slowly straighten arms to start position.

## Trainer's tips

- Depress your shoulder blades and contract your lats before you begin the pull-up.
- The higher percentage at which you set the machine, the more assistance you'll receive.
- Don't pull elbows behind you, drive them down toward the floor; this relieves any stress to the shoulders and keeps the challenge in your back.
- Don't lock elbows in start position, which adds stress to the elbow joints.
- Don't swing your body as you pull up or lower, because this decreases the exercise's effectiveness and compromises alignment.
- For more of a challenge, do this exercise unassisted (see page 88).

# Bent-Over Barbell Row INTERMEDIATE/ADVANCED

***Muscles Worked:*** *latissimus dorsi, teres major, rear deltoid; rhomboids and middle trapezius as stabilizers; biceps assist pulling action*

## Technique

1. Standing with legs hip-width apart, hold a barbell with an overhand grip, hands separated slightly wider than shoulder width and arms extended so barbell hangs in front of thighs.
2. Contract abdominal muscles to bring spine to a neutral position, and squeeze shoulder blades together. Bending knees slightly, flex forward from hips until torso is parallel to floor and forms one line from head to hips. Arms are extended in line with shoulders so barbell hangs down in front of shins, wrists straight.
3. Maintain position, and contract lats, bending elbows to pull the bar up toward rib cage.
4. Pause, then straighten arms to start position without changing position of your torso.

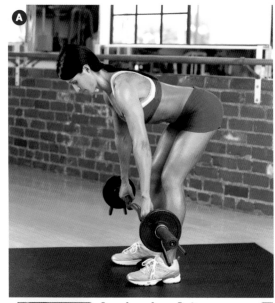


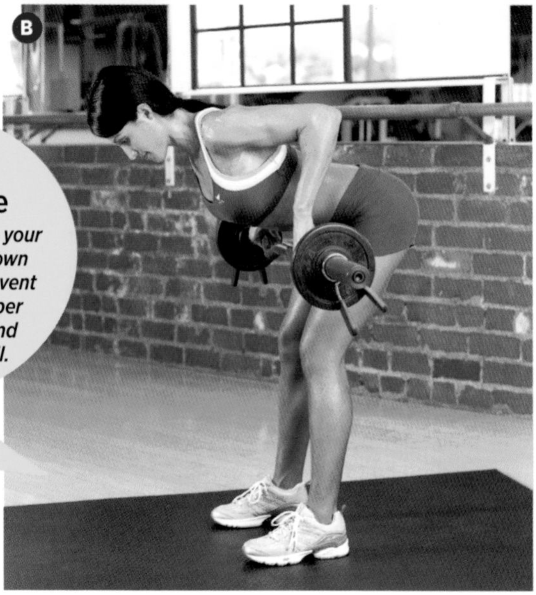


## Trainer's tips

- Keep abs contracted and chest lifted to maintain torso stability. If you can't sustain the position, lighten the load.
- Don't lift or pull up on your torso as you lift the bar; maintain the bent-over, parallel back position, keeping back muscles lengthened, head and neck aligned with spine.
- Drive up and back with your elbows so they move backwards as you pull the bar upward.
- Initiate the pulling action with your back muscles, and raise your elbows as high as possible in the top position.

### Inside Edge

***Continually squeeze your shoulder blades down and together to prevent rounding your upper back as you lift and lower the barbell.***

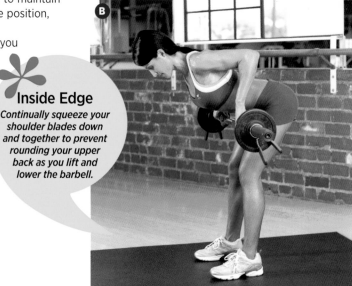

# High-Cable Row on Ball

INTERMEDIATE/ADVANCED

***Muscles Worked:*** *latissimus dorsi, teres major, rear deltoid; lower trapezius; rhomboids, middle trapezius as stabilizers; biceps assist pulling action*

## Technique

1. Attach a single handle to a high-cable pulley machine. Grasp it with a neutral grip, then sit erect on a stability ball positioned close enough to machine to extend arm in front of you at shoulder height, wrist straight. Place other hand on thigh.
2. Feet are on floor, hip-width apart, knees aligned over ankles.
3. Staying erect, squeeze shoulder blades back and down and contract abdominal muscles to maintain a neutral spine.
4. Maintaining position, balance and bend elbow back and in toward waist, aligning elbows with shoulders.
5. Extend arm to start position without changing torso position.

## Trainer's tips

- Before beginning the exercise, draw your scapulae down to stabilize your torso position.
- Keep your wrist straight and neutral so you focus on using your back muscles, not pulling with your arms.
- If you feel your shoulders roll forward or hunch up, lighten your weight.
- Keep your torso motionless so you're not rocking with the row.
- For variety, use an underhand grip or do the exercise two-handed, using a long bar or a rope attachment.
- To make this exercise easier, replace the ball with a flat bench.

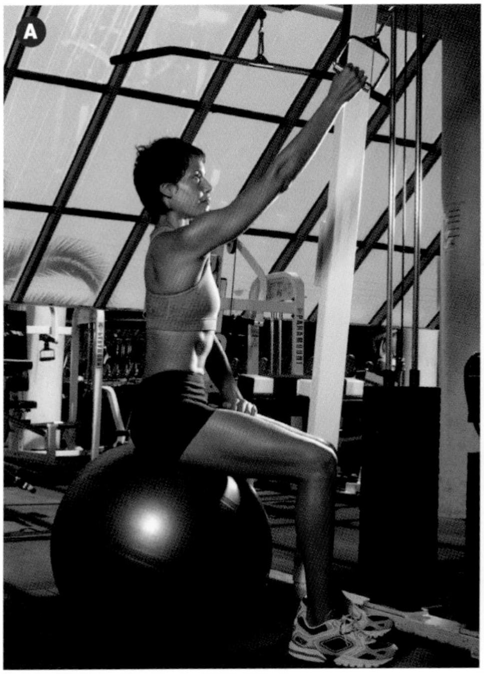

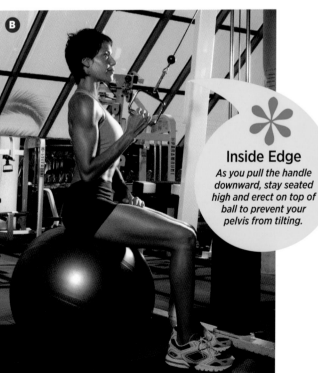


**Inside Edge**

***As you pull the handle downward, stay seated high and erect on top of ball to prevent your pelvis from tilting.***

# Lat Pulldown

BEGINNER/ INTERMEDIATE/ADVANCED

***Muscles Worked:*** *latissimus dorsi, teres major, lower fibers of trapezius; rhomboids and middle trapezius as stabilizers; biceps assist pulling action*

## Technique

1. Attach a long bar to a high-cable pulley. Taking an overhand grip on bar slightly wider than shoulder width, sit down and position thighs under the pads. Keep feet flat on floor, knees bent and in line with ankles.
2. Lean entire torso slightly back from your hips, positioning the bar in line with your breastbone, arms straight, wrists neutral.
3. Contract your abdominal muscles, keeping chest lifted and shoulder blades drawn down and together. Keep neck in neutral position.
4. Bend elbows down and in toward waist, aligning elbows with shoulders, pulling bar toward your upper chest as you lift chest toward the bar.
5. Pause, then straighten arms to start position.

## Trainer's tips

- Contract your lat muscles before bending your elbows so you can initiate the movement from your back, not your biceps.
- Keep your torso lifted for the entire move; don't collapse your torso as you pull the bar down.
- When releasing the bar, allow your arms to fully straighten and your back muscles to stretch before pulling the bar back down.
- Do not lean so far back that you place stress on your spine; lean back only enough to align bar with your upper chest. Neck remains neutral.
- For variety, do this exercise with a reverse grip (arms shoulder-width apart), or try different attachments, such as an angled V-bar or rope.

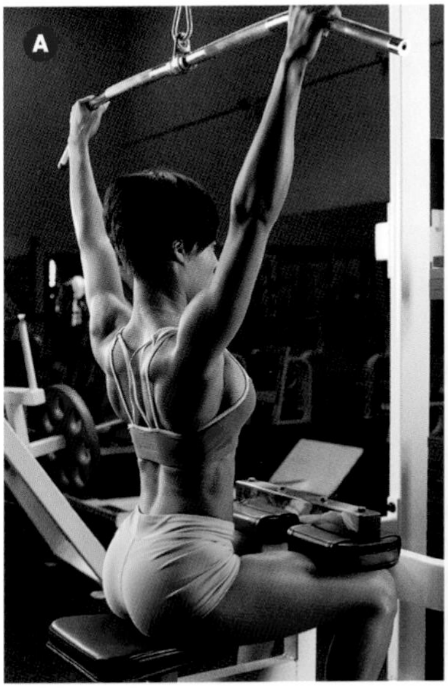


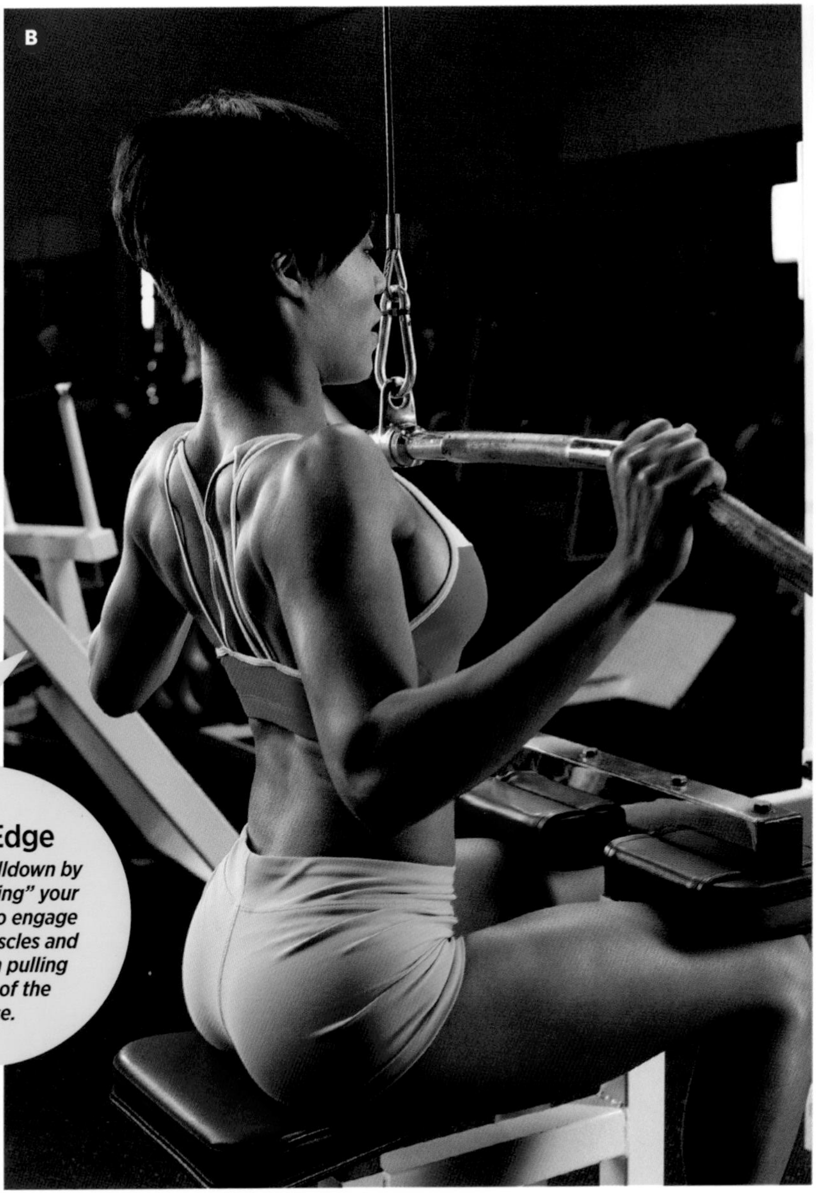


**Inside Edge**

*Initiate the pulldown by "pre-contracting" your lats in order to engage your back muscles and take any arm pulling action out of the exercise.*

# One-Arm Dumbbell Row

BEGINNER/INTERMEDIATE

***Muscles Worked:*** *latissimus dorsi, teres major, rear deltoid, lower fibers of trapezius; rhomboids and middle trapezius as stabilizers; biceps assist pulling action*

## Technique

1. Placing left hand and left knee on a flat bench, hinge forward from hips until back is parallel to floor. Head and neck are aligned with spine, right foot is on floor in line with left hip, knee slightly bent.
2. Hold a dumbbell in your right hand, arm extended directly in line with right shoulder, palm facing in.
3. Contract your abdominal muscles, squeezing shoulder blades down and together and keeping shoulders and hips square.
4. Keeping elbow close to your side, bend your elbow, bringing the dumbbell up and back toward lower ribs without rotating shoulders.
5. Pause, then straighten arm to start position. Do all reps and switch sides.

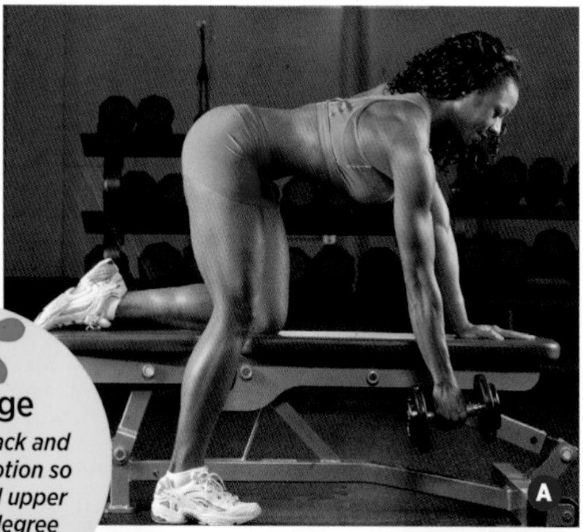


**Inside Edge**

***Move your arm back and up in one fluid motion so your forearm and upper arm form a 90-degree angle in the finish position.***

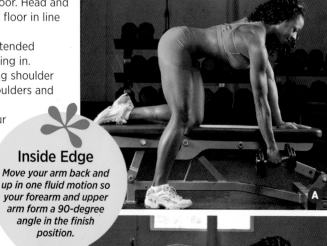

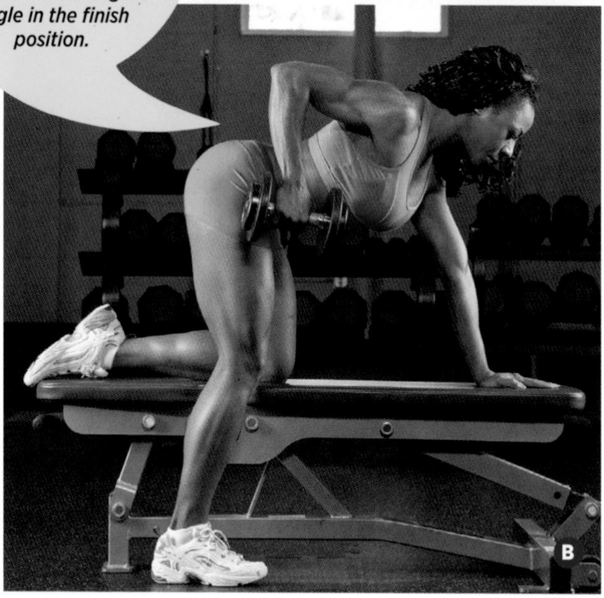


## Trainer's tips

- Keep your torso motionless; don't rotate your shoulders or hips.
- As you return to start position, let your shoulder blade slide forward.
- Use your abs to keep torso from sagging and to stabilize your position. Keep torso parallel to the floor.
- Pre-contract your lats with a small squeeze; concentrate on rowing with your lats, not your biceps.
- Begin by aligning your arm with your shoulder. This ensures proper mechanics and makes it easier to engage the lats.
- Don't round your shoulders or lift your elbow too high; this decreases the lat work and places stress on your neck and upper-back muscles.

# One-Arm Seated Cable Row

BEGINNER/INTERMEDIATE

***Muscles Worked:*** *latissimus dorsi, teres major, rear deltoid; rhomboids and middle trapezius as stabilizers; biceps assist pulling action*

## Technique

1. Attach a single handle to a low-cable pulley machine, then sit erect on bench, feet on support plate and separated hip-width apart, knees slightly bent, toes pointing up.
2. Hinging forward from hips, grasp handle with right hand, placing left hand on thigh. Sit erect with right arm extended at chest height, palm facing in.
3. Contract abdominal muscles to bring spine to neutral, and draw shoulder blades down and together.
4. Maintaining position, bend right elbow back and toward rib cage, keeping shoulders and hips square.
5. Straighten arm, returning to start position. Repeat for reps, then switch arms.

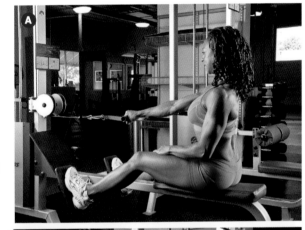

A

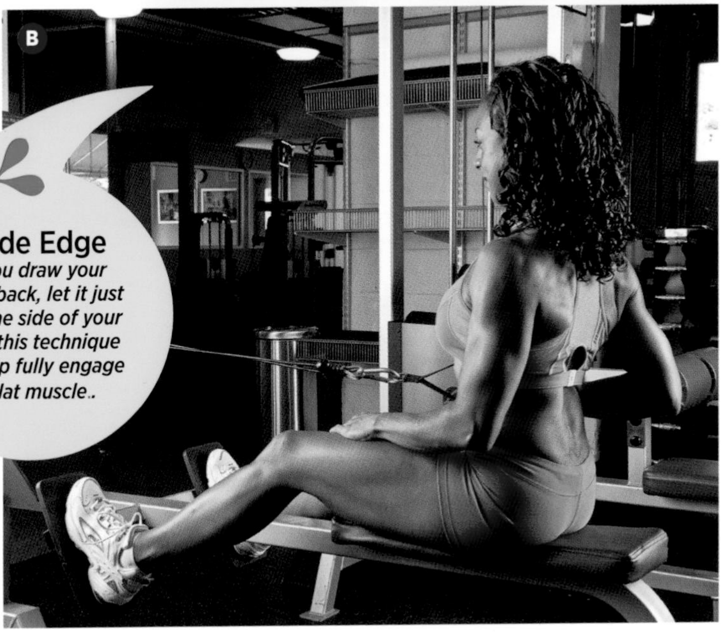

B

## Trainer's tips

- Use a weight that allows you to maintain an erect torso throughout the entire exercise without pulling you forward as you straighten arm or backwards as you pull.
- Keep shoulder blades drawn down and back to stabilize your upper back.
- Keep the handle at mid-abdomen height, as if drawing a straight line back from the machine as you row.
- Keep your wrist neutral or straight; cocking your wrist places strain on your forearm muscles.

**Inside Edge**

***As you draw your elbow back, let it just skim the side of your torso; this technique will help fully engage the lat muscle..***

# Pull-Up ADVANCED

***Muscles Worked:** latissimus dorsi, teres major, rear deltoids; rhomboids, middle trapezius, abdominals and erector spinae as stabilizers; biceps assist pulling action*

## Technique

1. Grasp a pull-up bar with an overhand grip, hands slightly wider than shoulder-width apart. Let your body hang, knees bent and aligned with hips, ankles crossed. Shoulders and hips are stacked, arms straight.
2. Contract your abdominal muscles to help maintain a motionless body without flexing your hips or overarching your spine.
3. Squeezing your scapulae down and together, focus on contracting your lats as you bend your elbows, driving them down toward your sides to pull your body up, lifting your chest up toward the bar.
4. Pause, then slowly lower your body by fully straightening your arms, being cautious not to let your body swing or your back arch.

## Trainer's tips

- Always start from a full hanging position with arms straight, rather than keeping your elbows bent at the bottom.
- Try not to use your arms to help with the initial pull; this takes the emphasis away from the back.
- Beginners should practice good pull-up form by: learning on a gravity-assisted machine, standing on a low bench to get into position, and doing partial pull-ups or having a spotter assist in the final phase of the movement.
- If you're advanced, try draping a thick rope over the bar and doing your pull-ups while grasping the rope. The instability of the rope will challenge your neuromuscular system and your grip will improve tremendously.

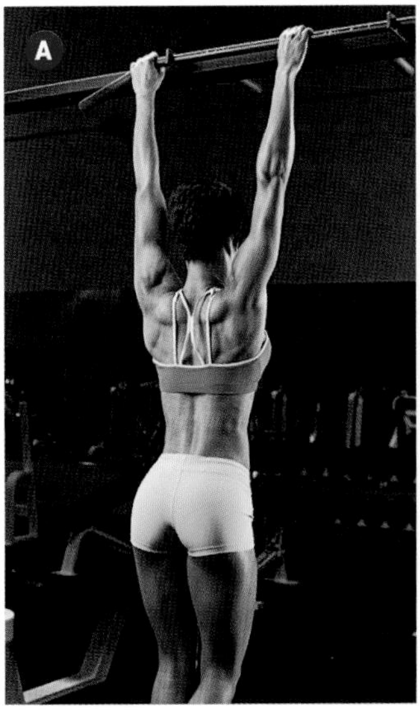


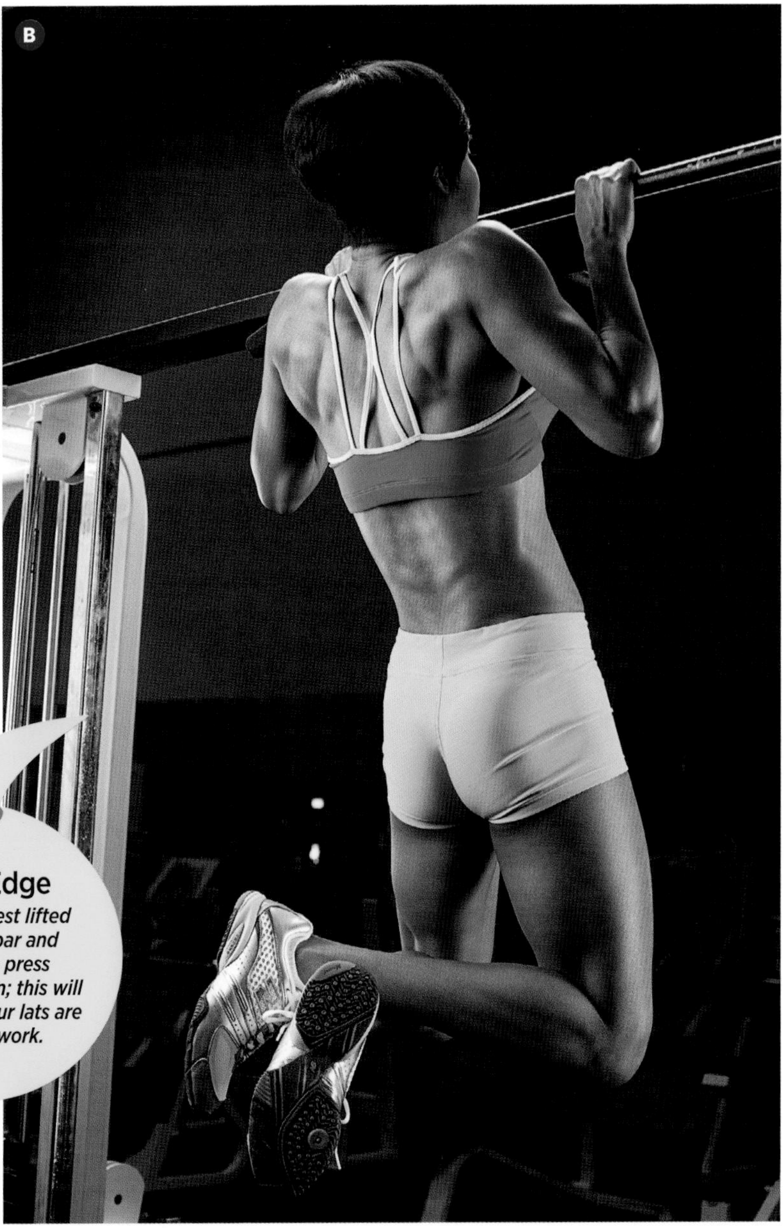


### Inside Edge

*Keep your chest lifted toward the bar and continue to press shoulders down; this will help ensure your lats are doing the work.*

# Seated Cable Row INTERMEDIATE/ADVANCED

***Muscles Worked:** latissimus dorsi, teres major, rear deltoids; rhomboids and middle trapezius as stabilizers; biceps assist pulling action*

## Technique

1. Attach a close-grip parallel handle to a cable row pulley, then sit erect on bench with feet on support plate, separated hip-width apart, knees slightly bent and toes pointing up.
2. Hinge forward from hips and grasp the handle with both hands, then sit erect with arms extended at chest height, palms facing in.
3. Contract abdominal muscles to bring spine to a neutral position, and draw shoulder blades down and together.
4. Maintain position and bend elbows back and toward rib cage, keeping arms close to the sides of your torso until handle just touches rib cage, elbows behind you.
5. Slowly straighten arms to start position without releasing upper-back muscles.

## Trainer's tips

- Don't jerk your body backwards to complete the movement; keep your torso vertical and erect for both the pulling and releasing phases.
- The rowing motion should come from the upper back.
- Keep your chest lifted, shoulders down and back throughout the exercise; avoid lifting your shoulders up toward your ears as you start to pull.
- If you have a hard time keeping your torso upright, have a spotter put her knee on the bench directly behind your back so your entire torso is lightly touching her thigh, then maintain this position.
- Experiment with different attachments and grips to vary your workout and the muscular emphasis.

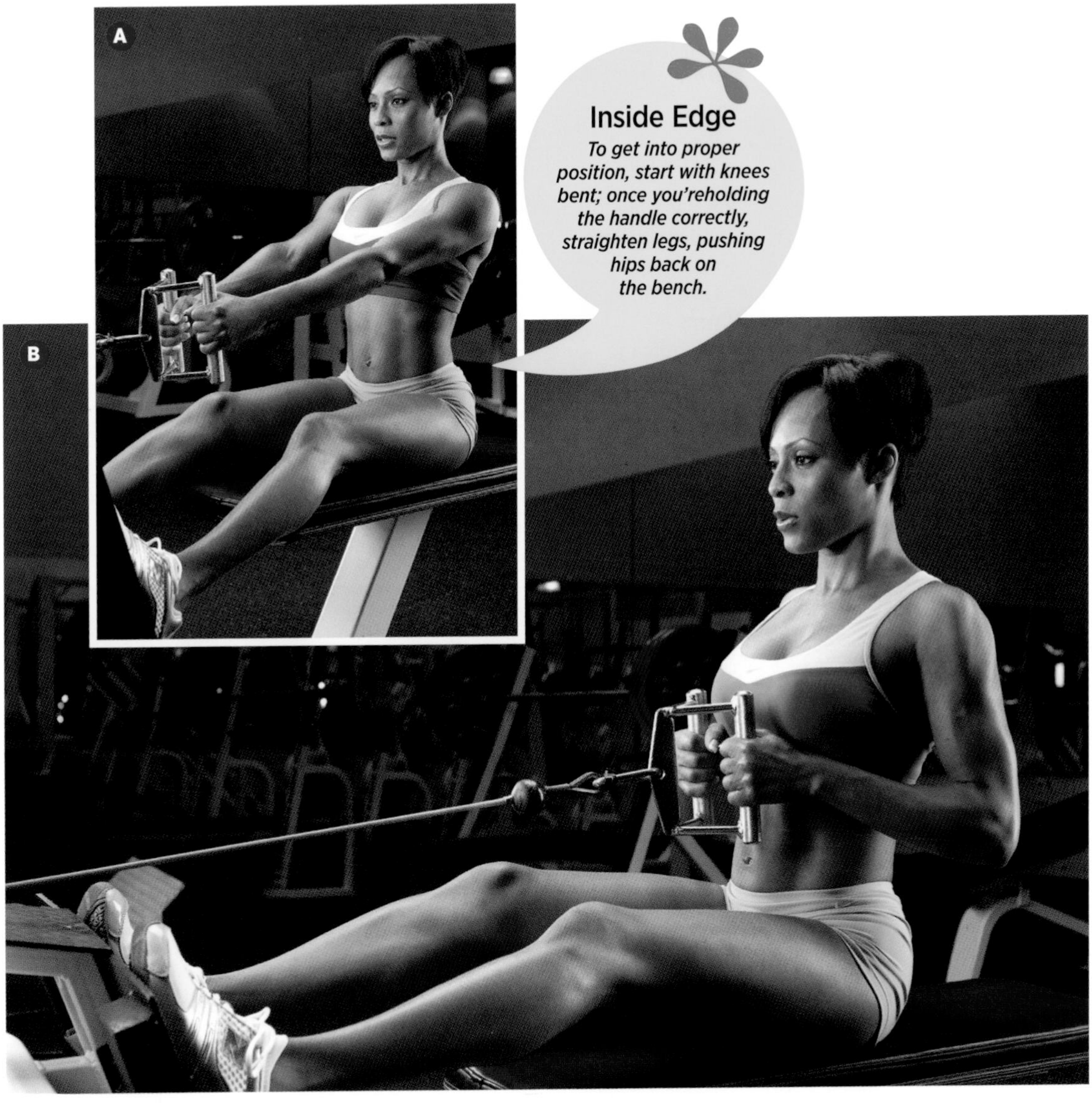


**Inside Edge**

*To get into proper position, start with knees bent; once you'reholding the handle correctly, straighten legs, pushing hips back on the bench.*

# Smith Machine Incline Row ADVANCED

***Muscles Worked:*** *latissimus dorsi, teres major, rear deltoids; rhomboids, middle trapezius, abdominals, erector spinae and gluteus maximus as stabilizers; biceps assist pulling action*

## Technique

1. Adjust bar of a Smith machine to rib-cage height when standing. Grasp bar with an underhand grip, hands slightly wider than shoulder-width apart and walk feet out in front of you so legs are extended and together to balance on heels. Arms are extended so bar is directly over upper rib cage.
2. Contract abdominal muscles to bring spine to neutral. Hang with head, neck, torso and legs forming one straight line from head to heels.
3. Maintaining body position, bend elbows to pull yourself up toward bar; lead with your chest and don't strain your neck.
4. Slowly straighten arms, lowering to start position without sagging torso.

## Trainer's tips

- The best way to get in the proper position is to first align the bar over your rib cage, then walk feet outward. You may have to make minor adjustments once you're in hanging position.
- In the final position, your elbows will be aligned with shoulders just as they would for any other type of seated row.
- Keep chest lifted toward the bar and lift your entire body as one unit so your hips don't drag. Contract your glutes and leg muscles to help stabilize your position and maintain the inverted plank position.
- For an easier version, do this exercise with knees bent at 90 degrees and aligned over ankles.

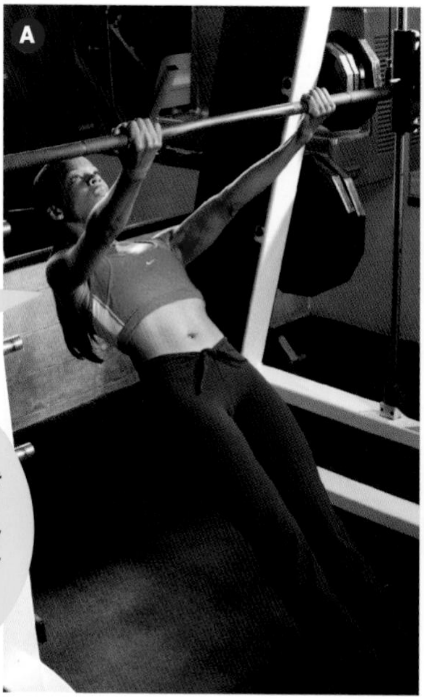


**Inside Edge**

***Align bar between chest and upper rib cage; if your shoulders hunch or bar comes too far under your chin, re-establish your position.***

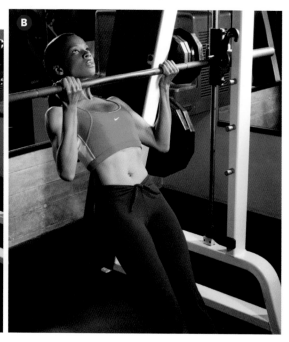

# Machine Row BEGINNER

***Muscles Worked:*** *upper fibers of latissimus dorsi, teres major, lower fibers of trapezius; rhomboids and middle trapezius as stabilizers*

## Technique

1. Sit on a row machine and adjust seat so the support pad is at chest height. Arms are parallel to the floor when extended, knees bent and in line with ankles, feet flat on floor or resting on foot plates.
2. Grasping handles and keeping arms straight, lean torso lightly against support pad without collapsing rib cage.
3. Contract abdominal muscles so spine is neutral, shoulder blades drawn down and together, chest lifted, shoulders relaxed.
4. Maintain torso position and contract lat muscles first, then bend elbows out and keep elbows wide. With wrists neutral, torso erect, pull until elbows are even with torso.
5. Pause, then extend arms to start position without rounding back or shoulders.

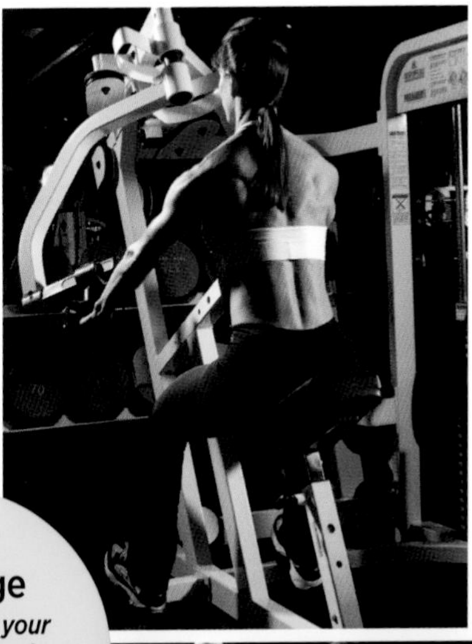

**Inside Edge**

***Think of drawing your elbows out and back, rather than straight back; this will keep the lats engaged and your shoulders down.***

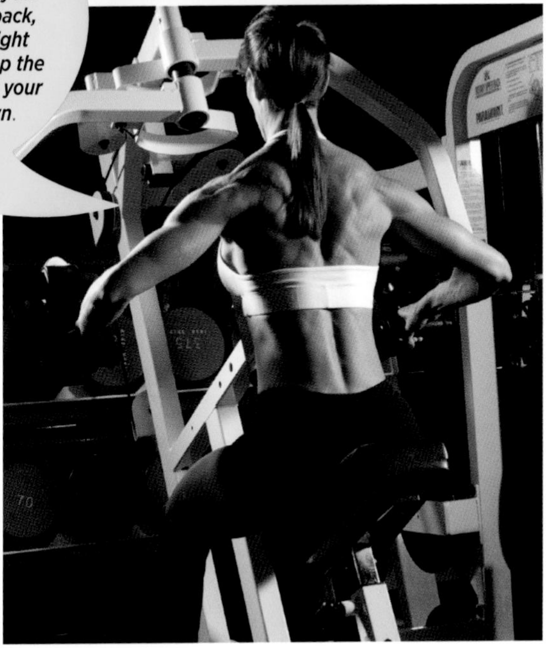

## Trainer's tips

- Position is important: If your seat is too high or too far from the stack, you'll hunch your shoulders or be forced to lean too heavily on the support pad.
- Use enough weight to challenge your muscles, but not so much that you can't bring elbows all the way back.
- Keep shoulder blades depressed and retracted to sustain an erect position.
- Keep torso lightly in contact with support pad; even in the final position, it should still be touching the pad.
- For variety, change or alternate grips, or superset with a lat pulldown.
- For more of a challenge, lighten weight and perform single-handedly.

## Beginner Workouts

***Directions:** This is a progressive six-week program using moderate weight. Do the exercises listed twice a week.*

| WEEK | EXERCISE | SETS | REPS |
|---|---|---|---|
| 1 & 2 | Assisted Pull-Up | 1–2 | 12–15 |
| | Machine Row | 1–2 | 8–12 |
| 3 & 4 | Lat Pulldown | 2 | 10–12 |
| | One-Arm Dumbbell Row | 2 | 10–12 |
| 5 & 6 | Warm-up: Assisted Pull-Up | 1 | 12–15 |
| | Lat Pulldown or Machine Row | 2 | 8–12 |
| | One-Arm Dumbbell Row | 2 | 10–12 |

**Notes**

*Rest 45–60 seconds between sets. At the end of six weeks, progress to intermediate workouts if you're ready.*

## Intermediate Workouts

***Directions:** This is a progressive six-week program using moderate weight. Do the exercises twice per week. For lighter or heavier weight, adjust reps..*

| WEEK | EXERCISE | SETS | REPS |
|---|---|---|---|
| 1 & 2 | Assisted Pull-Up | 2–3 | 10–15 |
| | Seated Cable Row (Drop set)* | 2 | 10/5 |
| | Bent-Over Barbell Row | 2–3 | 8–12 |
| 3 & 4 | Angled Pulldown | 1st** | 10–12 |
| | ***To pyramid sets, increase weight* | 2nd | 8–10 |
| | *as you decrease reps.* | 3rd | 6–8 |
| | One-Arm Seated Cable Row | 2 | 8–12 |
| | Assisted Pull-Up | 2 | 10–12 |
| | Bent-Over Barbell Row | 2–3 | 8–12 |
| 5 & 6 | ***Day 1 Workout*** | | |
| | Assisted Pull-Up | 2–3 | 10–12 |
| | Lat Pulldown | 2–3 | 10–12 |
| | Seated Cable Row | 2–3 | 8–12 |
| | Bent-Over Barbell Row | 2–3 | 10–15 |
| | ***Day 2 Workout*** | | |
| | High-Cable Row on Ball | 2–3 | 10–12 |
| | One-Arm Seated Cable Row | 2 | 8–12 |
| | One-Arm Dumbbell Row | 2 | 8–12 |

**Notes**

*Rest 45–60 seconds between sets. After six weeks, progress to advanced workouts if you're ready.*

**For drop sets, reduce weight enough to complete five additional reps.*

## Advanced Workouts

***Directions:*** ***Perform two workouts a week, choosing from the following programs. You can also do biceps work on the same day, or include it as part of a superset program.***

| EXERCISE | SETS | REPS |
|---|---|---|
| *Workout 1* | | |
| Lat Pulldown | 1st | 10–12 |
| (Increase weight | 2nd | 8–10 |
| as you decrease reps) | 3rd | 6–8 |
| Bent-Over Barbell Row | 3 | 8–10 |
| One-Arm Dumbbell Row | 3 | 10–12 |
| *Workout 2* | | |
| ***Drop set each set:**** | | |
| Angled Pulldown | 3 | 10/5 |
| One-Arm Seated Cable Row | 3 | 10–12 |
| One-Arm Dumbbell Row | 3 | 10–12 |
| Smith-Machine Incline Row | 2–3 | 8–10 |
| *Workout 3* | | |
| Pull-Up | 2–3 | 8–12 |
| High-Cable Row on Ball or Lat Pulldown | 2–3 | 8–12 |
| Seated Cable Row | 3 | 8–12 |

***Notes***

*Rest 60–90 seconds between sets.*
**For drop sets, reduce weight enough to complete five additional reps.*

## Can't-Get-to-the-Gym Workouts

***Directions:*** ***Do the following exercises when you want to work out at home, or on the road. For variety, change the order. You can do biceps work the same day, or as a superset with lats.***

| EXERCISE | SETS | REPS |
|---|---|---|
| One-Arm Dumbbell Row* | 2-3 | 8-15 |
| High-Cable Row on Ball (use a resistance tube in a doorjam) | 2-3 | 8-15 |
| Pull-Up (use a pull-up bar in a doorway) | 2-3 | 5-10 |
| Bent-Over Row (use a barbell or dumbbells) | 2-3 | 8-15 |

***Notes***

*Rest 60–90 seconds between sets. If you're a beginner, only do the exercises marked with an asterisk (*).*

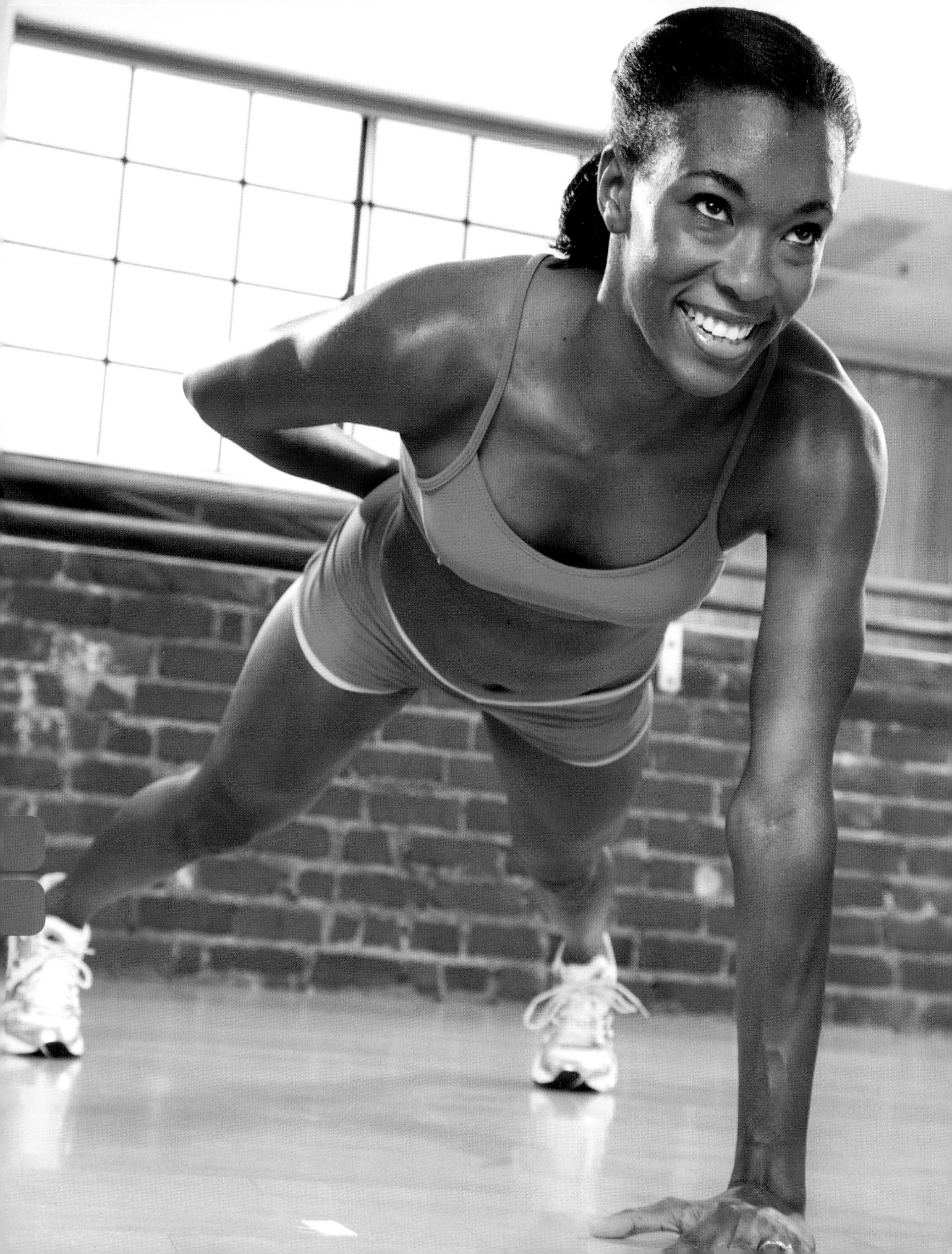

# Chapter 6

# Chest

*Lift your way to a strong, shapely chest.*

YOUR MAIN CHEST MUSCLE, THE PECTORALIS MAJOR, is a large, fan-shape muscle with multiple attachments. One portion attaches to the middle and inner part of your collarbone, working with the anterior deltoid (your front shoulder muscle) to move your arms forward and upward and rotate the arm inward. The other part attaches on your breastbone (sternum) and upper six ribs, and is stimulated only in downward and forward arm movements. Both portions attach together near the top of your upper arm bone. The serratus anterior, located on either side of your rib cage; and the pectoralis minor, a small muscle under the pectoralis major, both stabilize your shoulder blades as your arms move forward. The triceps are involved in any chest pushing motion.

## General Guidelines for *TRAINING CHEST*

***Finish with a peak contraction, squeezing at the top of the movement.***

To recruit muscle fibers throughout the entire range of motion, contract your pecs and continue to squeeze them through the entire press, flye or push-up. Finish the movement with a peak contraction, squeezing at the top of the movement.

Carefully monitor the depth of arm lowering. If elbows are too far below shoulder height, the return phase is initiated by the anterior deltoid instead of the pecs, which can be stressful to the shoulder muscles and connective tissue, and limit the amount of weight you can lift.

Balance chest work with upper-back exercises; these two opposing muscle groups easily go out of balance if chest muscles become too tight or if the upper back is weak, causing rounded shoulders and a slumped posture.

Rotate exercises in your routine regularly; different positions stimulate different parts of the pecs. Flat-bench exercises and standard push-up positions will target middle pec fibers; incline-bench exercises hone in on upper pec fibers; whereas decline-bench and standing cable exercises recruit more lower and outer pec fibers.

# Ball Push-Up on Shins INTERMEDIATE/ADVANCED

***Muscles Worked:*** *pectoralis major; anterior deltoids; triceps; abdominals, spine extensors, glutes as stabilizers*

## Technique

1. Lying facedown over a stability ball, place hands on floor in front of you and walk hands forward, rolling ball underneath you until you're balanced with the ball under your shins and ankles.
2. Keeping arms extended with fingertips facing forward, place hands slightly wider than shoulders.
3. Contract abdominal muscles, drawing tailbone down so your body forms one straight line from head to heels in "plank" position.
4. Maintain plank and bend elbows, lowering chest toward floor until elbows are in line with shoulders, wrists aligned under elbows with forearms parallel to each other.
5. Using chest and triceps, press back up to start position.

## Trainer's tips

- Avoid gripping the floor with hand and wrist muscles to compensate for the instability. Concentrate on proper shoulder and elbow alignment: Relax wrists and loosely spread fingers wide on floor.
- Don't let your head droop as you lower toward the floor; keep head and neck aligned with spine. Moving your head as you push up causes neck strain, and the additional movement can make balancing even harder.
- For more of a challenge, lift one foot off ball or place both hands on a stability tool such as an airex pad.
- For a high-intensity tri-set, follow push-ups with one-arm cable flye or single-arm pec-deck flye and a barbell bench press drop set.

### Inside Edge

***Good setup is key to this exercise. Make sure body is draped over center of ball at beginning, and shins stay centered as you roll forward.***

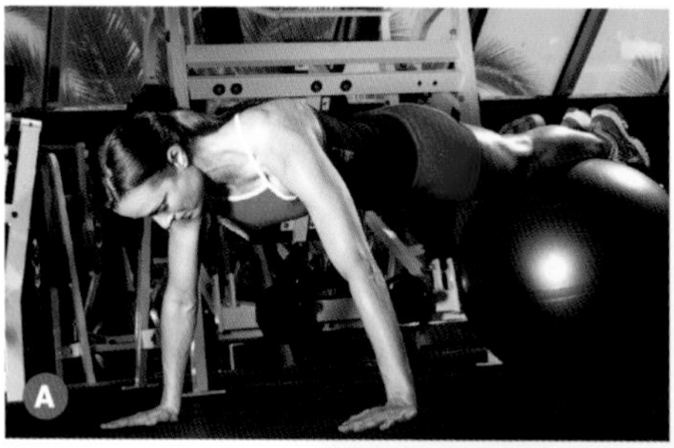
A

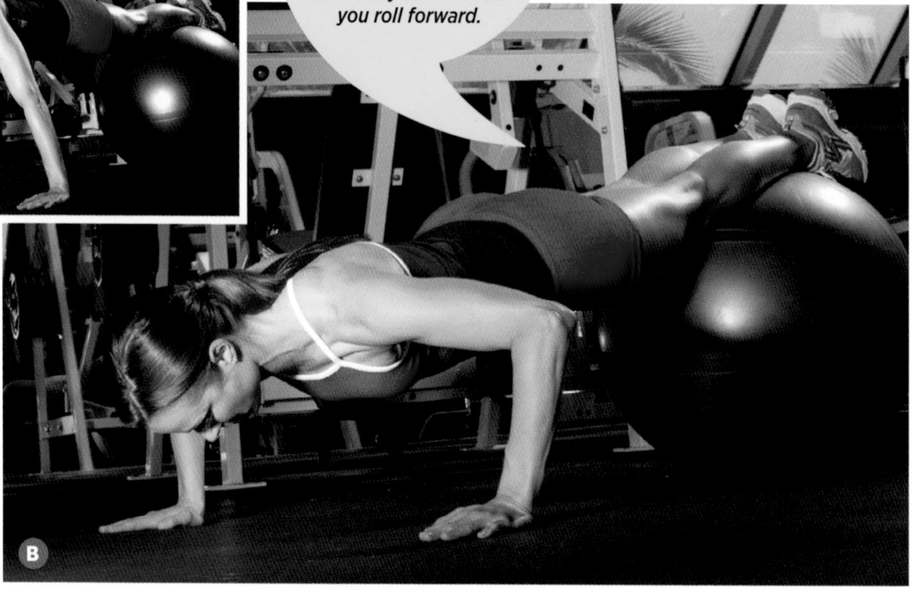
B

# Ball Push-Up on Thighs BEGINNER

***Muscles Worked:*** *pectoralis major; anterior deltoids; triceps; abdominals, spine extensors and glutes as stabilizers*

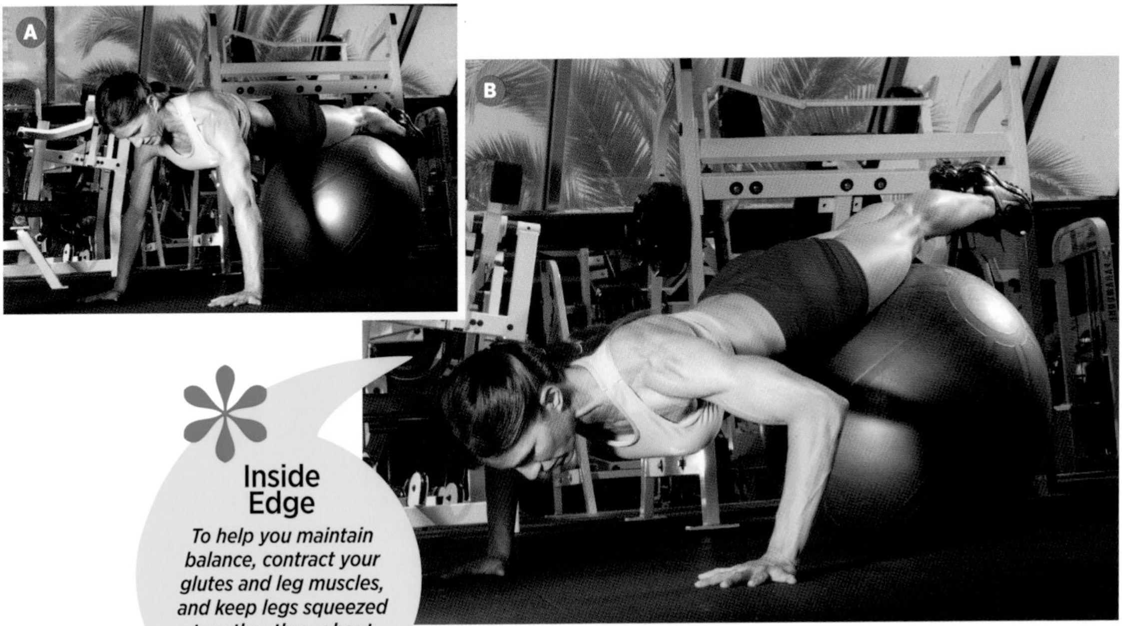


**Inside Edge**

***To help you maintain balance, contract your glutes and leg muscles, and keep legs squeezed together throughout the entire movement.***

## Technique

1. Lie facedown over a stability ball, placing hands on floor in front of you. Walk hands forward, rolling ball underneath you until you're balanced on the ball at your thighs, above kneecaps.
2. Keeping arms extended with fingertips facing forward, place hands slightly wider than shoulders.
3. Contract abdominal muscles, drawing tailbone down so your body forms one straight line from head to heels in "plank" position.
4. Maintain plank and bend elbows, lowering chest toward the floor until elbows are in line with shoulders, wrists aligned under elbows with forearms parallel to each other.
5. Using chest and triceps, press back up to start position.

## Trainer's tips

- Don't get so focused on the balancing that you forget about your form.
- To make the balancing easier, make sure your upper body is stable and shoulders are not in front of or behind your arms.
- Even though your legs are supported on the ball, it's easy to let your abs sag or to collapse your shoulder blades; both of these mistakes strain your shoulders and spine, and decrease the workload of your pecs and triceps.
- If you're not ready to advance to the ball push-up on the shins, gradually increase the difficulty of this one by lifting one leg off the ball.

# Barbell Bench Press INTERMEDIATE/ADVANCED

***Muscles Worked:*** *pectoralis major, anterior deltoids, triceps*

## Technique

1. Lying on a flat bench with knees bent and feet on the floor or edge of bench, hold a barbell with an overhand grip above midchest, arms straight but not locked, and slightly wider than shoulder-width apart.
2. Contract abdominal muscles so back is in a neutral position; squeeze shoulder blades together and down to stabilize your torso. Chest is lifted and shoulders are relaxed.
3. Bend elbows and lower bar toward chest until elbows are even with shoulders or slightly lower, wrists aligned over elbows.
4. Keep chest lifted as you contract chest and triceps muscles to straighten arms and drive bar up over chest without locking elbows.
5. Pause before lowering.

## Trainer's tips

- Focus more on pushing evenly rather than on pushing the bar up. If you notice one side is consistently weaker, supplement your workout with single-side exercises that force the weaker side to work.
- Don't lower the bar to a full stretch position, or so far below your shoulders that you can't press it back up.
- Don't cock wrists backwards, causing you to lose balance of the bar; keep wrists aligned over your elbows to ensure that you're using your chest and triceps to do the work.
- Use a spotter for drop sets. Set up the bar with several smaller plates and have a spotter quickly strip off one at a time on your last set.

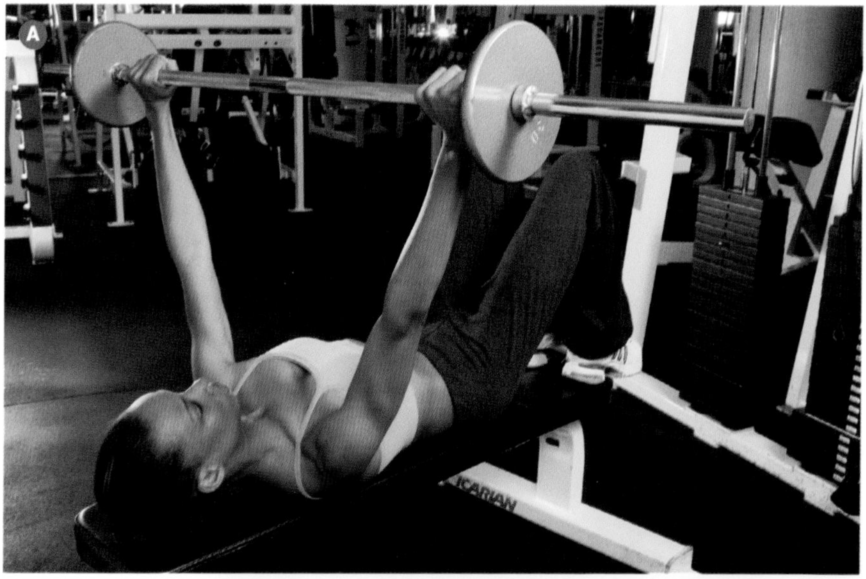


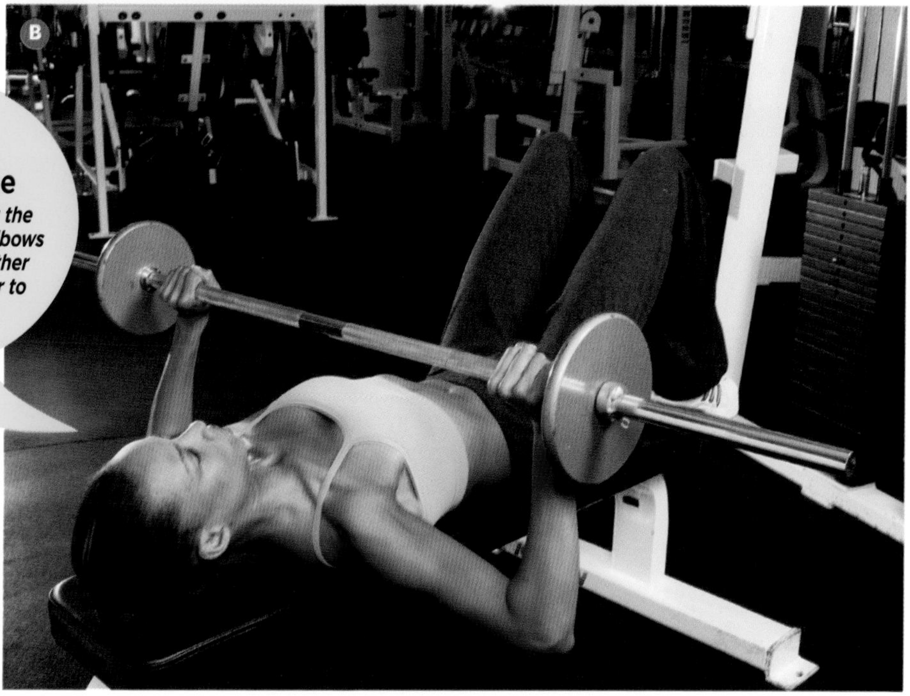


**Inside Edge**

***To avoid lowering the bar too far, align elbows and shoulders rather than bringing bar to touch chest.***

# Flat-Bench Dumbbell Flye

BEGINNER/INTERMEDIATE/ADVANCED

***Muscles Worked:*** *pectoralis major, anterior deltoid*

## Technique

1. Holding a dumbbell in each hand, lie faceup on a flat bench, knees bent and feet on the floor.
2. Extend arms directly above midchest, aligning arms with shoulders and keeping elbows slightly rounded, palms facing in, wrists neutral.
3. Contract abdominal muscles so spine is neutral, and squeeze your shoulder blades together and down to stabilize upper back.
4. Lower dumbbells in an arc-like pattern out and away from chest until elbows are aligned with shoulders and you feel a slight stretch across the front of your shoulders.
5. Contract chest muscles, driving dumbbells up and in to start position without changing angle at elbows.

## Trainer's tips

- Maintain a neutral position in both your spine and wrists. Overarching will reduce stability and make heavier weights more difficult to control; overflexing wrists can cause carpal-tunnel syndrome.
- Don't allow elbows to drop below shoulder height, which can stress the shoulder joint as well as overstretch pectoral connective tissue.
- For variety, use an incline bench or lower cables with single handles or ropes attached to each side. Place a bench between the weight stacks so lower cables align with shoulders.
- For more of a challenge, perform flyes with one arm, or lie on a stability ball instead of a bench.

### Inside Edge

***To maximize pec recruitment, focus on lifting and lowering in an arc motion, keeping elbow and wrist angles unchanged throughout the movement.***

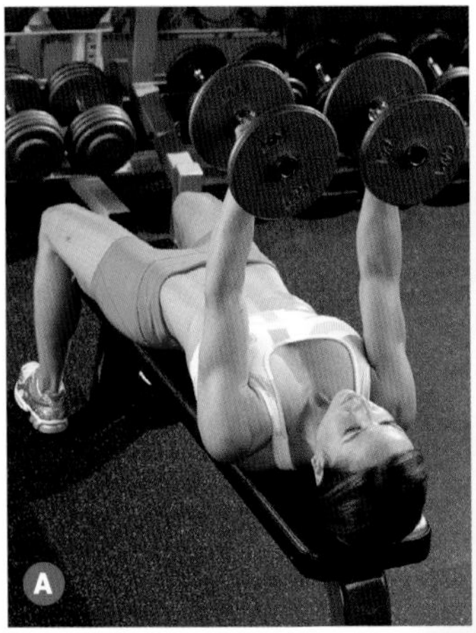
A

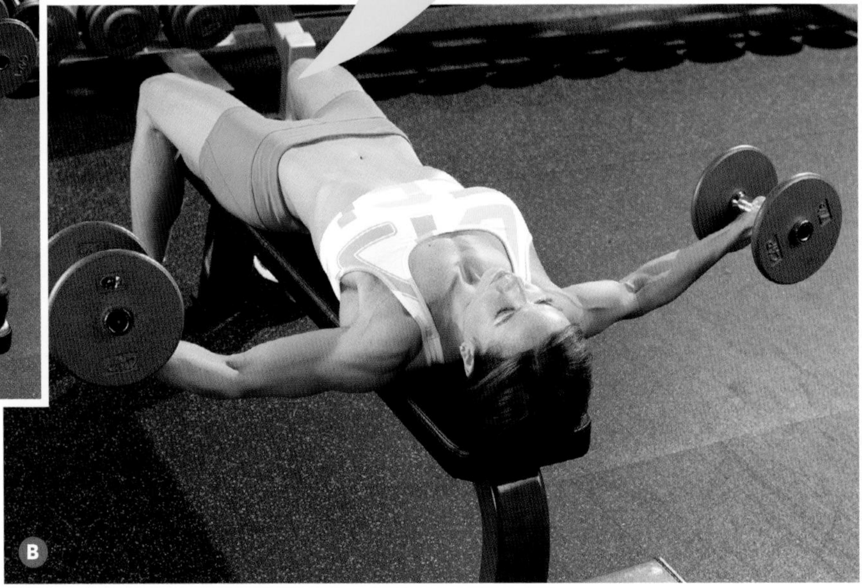
B

# Flat-Bench Dumbbell Press

BEGINNER/INTERMEDIATE/ADVANCED

***Muscles Worked:*** *pectoralis major, anterior deltoids, triceps*

## Technique

1. Grasp a pair of dumbbells and lie faceup on a flat bench, knees bent and feet on floor or edge of bench.
2. Raise arms straight up, aligned over the middle chest, palms facing forward, wrists neutral with dumbbells almost touching.
3. Contract abdominal muscles so spine is in a neutral position; squeeze shoulder blades together and down to stabilize your upper back.
4. Bend elbows, lowering dumbbells down and out toward the sides of your chest until upper arms align with shoulders, elbows are bent at 90 degrees, wrists in line with elbows.
5. Contract chest and triceps to straighten arms, driving dumbbells up and in toward center of chest without locking elbows.

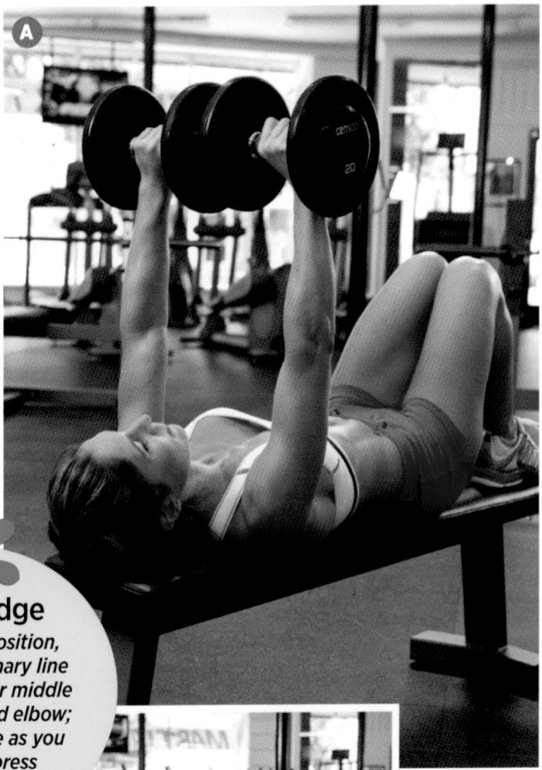
A

## Trainer's tips

- Avoid arching lower back, especially as you lower the weights; it won't help you and may cause injury, especially with heavier weights.
- Keeping shoulder blades drawn together, even at the top of the movement, will stabilize the shoulders. This allows you to move more weight as well as keep the pecs engaged through the entire range of motion.
- For variety, lie on an incline bench or use an EZ-bar or barbell; you may be able to use heavier weight with a single bar, as it's more stable to lift than two dumbbells. Make sure to use a spotter when going heavy.
- For advanced training, compound set with dumbbell flyes.

**Inside Edge**

***To maintain position, draw an imaginary line connecting your middle finger, wrist and elbow; follow that line as you lower and press dumbbells back up.***

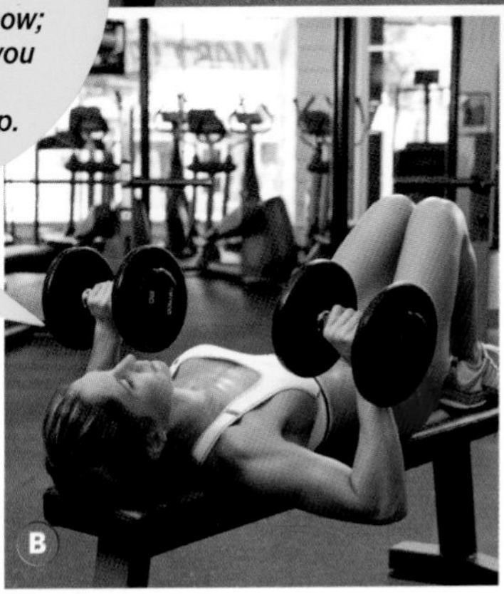
B

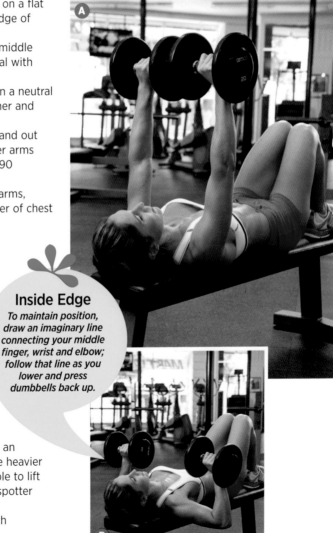

# Full Push-Up

INTERMEDIATE/ADVANCED

***Muscles Worked:*** *pectoralis major; anterior deltoids; triceps; abdominals spine extensors, glutes as stabilizers.*

## Technique

1. Kneel on all fours, arms straight and slightly wider than shoulder-width apart, wrists in line with your shoulders, fingers facing forward, knees in line with hips.
2. Contract abdominal muscles so back is in neutral, and squeeze shoulder blades together and down.
3. Extend one leg at a time behind you so you're supported on the balls of your feet and your body forms a straight line from head to heels; look straight down with neck extended.
4. Bend elbows out to sides, lowering torso toward floor until elbows are bent at 90 degrees and aligned with shoulders.
5. Straighten arms, pressing back up to start position without locking elbows.

## Trainer's tips

- With the longer lever of a full push-up, more attention needs to be paid to alignment. Anterior shoulder pain is a sure sign to assess your upper-arm alignment and make the necessary adjustments.
- Keep head and neck aligned with spine throughout the entire exercise.
- It's not necessary to bring your chest to the floor. If you have long arms, lowering too far will take elbows beyond 90 degrees, stressing shoulder and elbow joints, and making it difficult to recover and press your body back up.
- For a greater challenge, perform the push-up with a balance tool under feet or hands, or with feet elevated on a bench or stability ball.

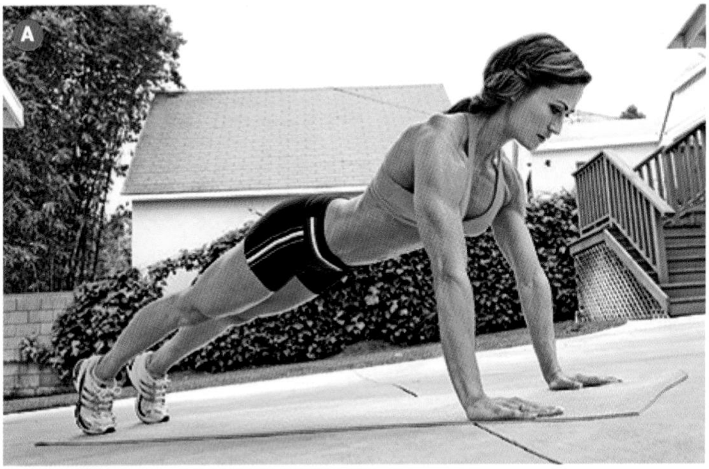

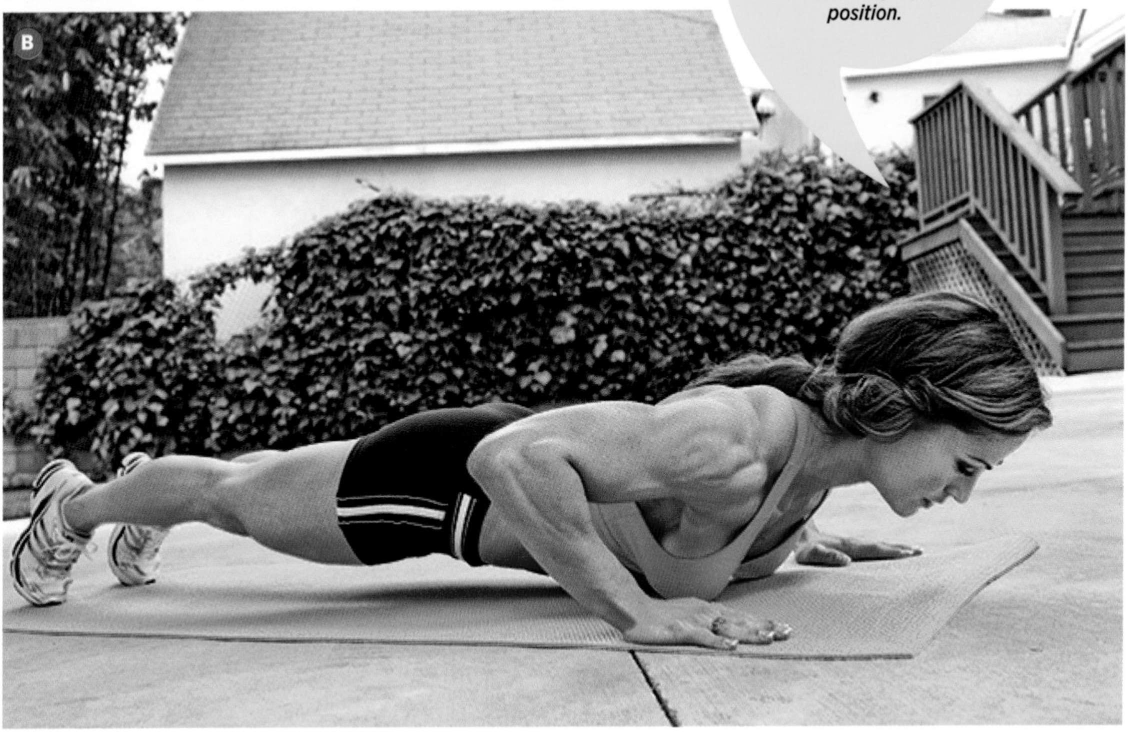

## Inside Edge

*To keep abs and hips from sagging at the bottom, contract your glutes and leg muscles to maintain a tight plank position.*

# Incline Dumbbell Press

BEGINNER/INTERMEDIATE/ADVANCED

***Muscles Worked:** pectoralis major, with emphasis on upper fibers; anterior deltoid; triceps*

## Technique

1. Holding a dumbbell in each hand, lie faceup on an incline bench adjusted to about 30–45 degrees. Feet are flat on floor shoulder-width apart, knees are bent and aligned over ankles.
2. Press dumbbells up overhead to a vertical position above upper chest, arms straight but not locked, palms facing forward.
3. Contract abdominal muscles so spine is neutral, and squeeze shoulder blades together and down.
4. Bend elbows, lowering dumbbells down and out to sides of chest until elbows are aligned with shoulders and bent at 90 degrees, wrists over elbows.
5. Straighten arms, driving dumbbells up and in above center of chest without locking elbows.

## Trainer's tips:

- To ensure the proper arc of movement, start with arms completely vertical at the top of the movement, then move them down and out. If you start with arms too far forward, the front delts will tire and be unable to stabilize properly.
- Although you may be tempted to lower elbows below the shoulders at the bottom of the movement to feel the stretch, you're actually risking injury to the fairly unstable shoulder joint if you exceed the range of motion.
- For variety, use a flat bench or barbell, or perform with one arm at a time.
- For more of a core challenge, place both feet on a stability ball.

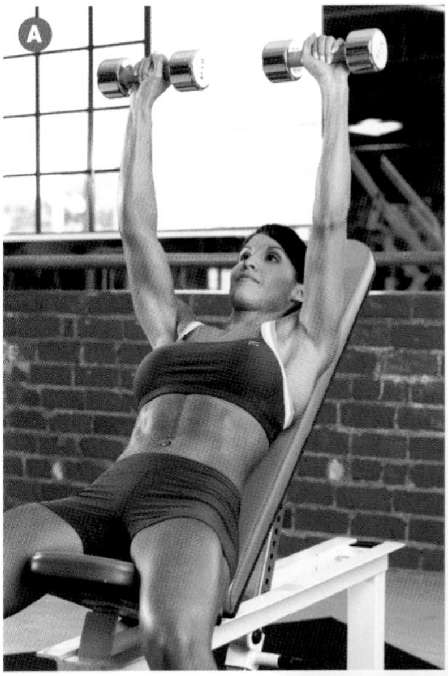


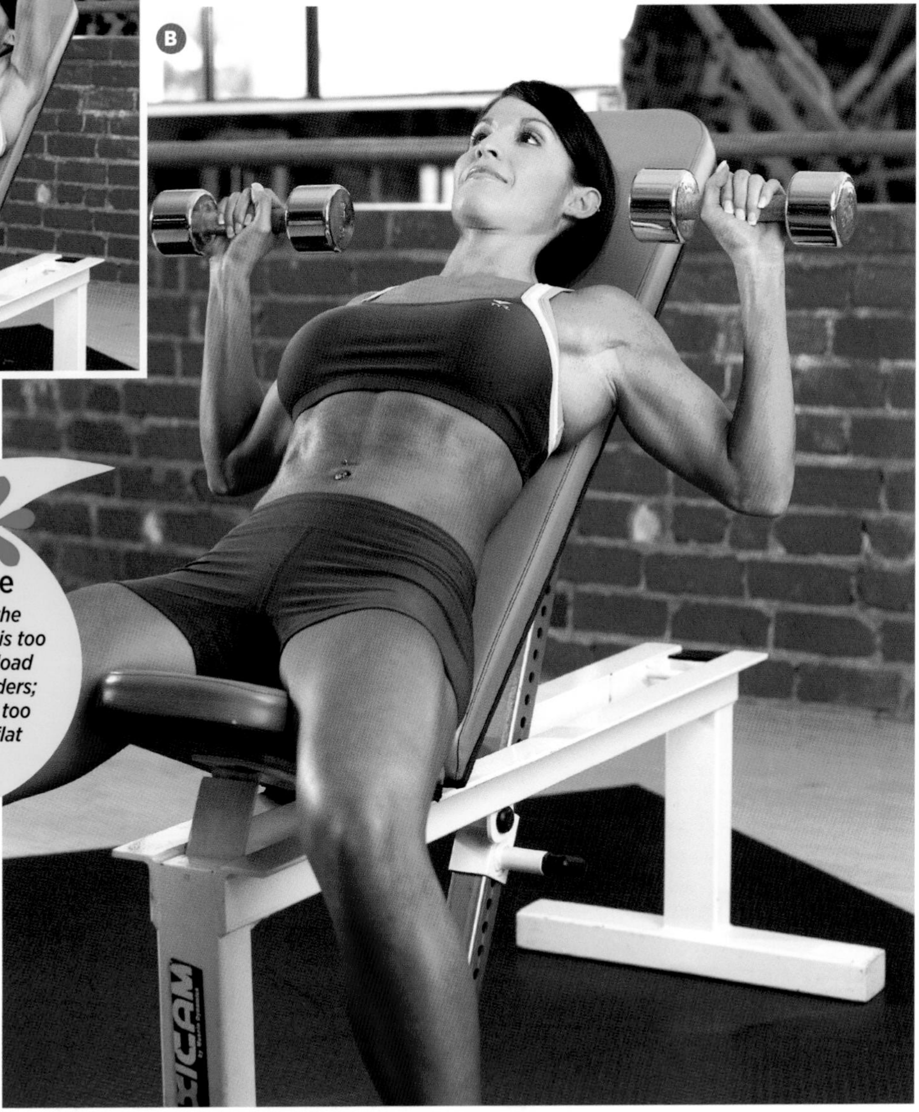


## Inside Edge

*Properly adjust the bench. If seat back is too upright, the workload shifts to the shoulders; if the seat back is too low, it mimics a flat bench.*

# Incline Low-Cable Flye ADVANCED

***Muscles Worked:** pectoralis major, with emphasis on the upper fibers; anterior deltoids*

## Technique

1. Adjust an incline bench to a 30–45-degree angle and position it equally between two low cables with single handles attached.
2. Sit on bench, knees bent and feet flat on floor. Grasp handles and lie back on bench, aligning handles over upper chest with elbows bent in a soft arc and knuckles almost touching, wrists neutral.
3. Contract abdominal muscles so spine is neutral, and squeeze shoulder blades together and down, chest lifted.
4. Keeping elbows in an arc and wrists neutral, open arms down and out to your sides until elbows are even with shoulders.
5. Contract chest muscles, bringing arms back up in an arc toward center of your chest.

## Trainer's tips

- Keep shoulder blades pulled back throughout the entire range of motion, rather than letting your back completely release as cables approach top of movement.
- Don't set the bench angle too high; it shifts the workload to the shoulders.
- Fight the urge to assist your chest muscles by bending the elbows or wrists more as you bring handles up. Keeping the angle at the elbows constant forces the pecs to do the work.
- For variety, substitute a stability ball for the bench. Walk feet out and drop hips to approximately the same torso angle as if you were using an incline bench.
- For more of a challenge, perform as a single-arm flye.

### Inside Edge

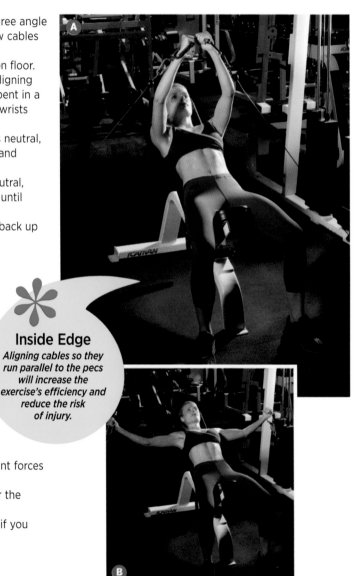

***Aligning cables so they run parallel to the pecs will increase the exercise's efficiency and reduce the risk of injury.***

# Knee Push-Up BEGINNER

***Muscles Worked:*** *pectoralis major; anterior deltoids; triceps; abdominals, spine extensors, glutes as stabilizers*

## Technique

1. Kneel on all fours, arms straight and in line with shoulders, knees under hips.
2. Walk hands forward about 6 inches, then press hips forward until body forms a straight line from head to hips. Separate hands so they're slightly wider than shoulder-width apart, fingers facing forward.
3. Contract abdominal muscles so spine is in a neutral position, and draw shoulder blades together and down.
4. Maintaining position, bend elbows out to sides, lowering torso toward the floor until elbows are bent at 90 degrees and aligned with shoulders.
5. Contract chest and triceps muscles to straighten arms and return to start position without locking elbows at the top.

## Trainer's tips

- If you experience lower back discomfort, align knees underneath hips, rather than behind them, and maintain this angle.
- Initiate the push-up using your chest and triceps; your abs should never sag and touch the floor.
- To avoid stressing the shoulder joint, keep elbows aligned straight out from shoulders and wrists.
- As soon as you feel strong enough, switch to the full push-up. The longer lever makes the exercise more difficult, making the pecs work harder.
- For a quick home workout, superset knee push-ups and bench dips. Rest between sets and repeat twice more.

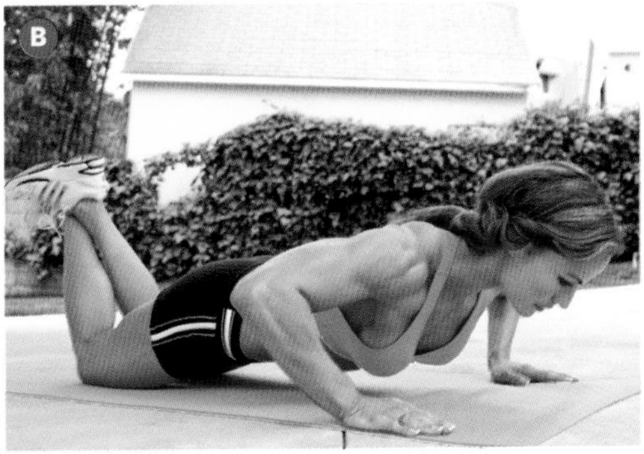
B

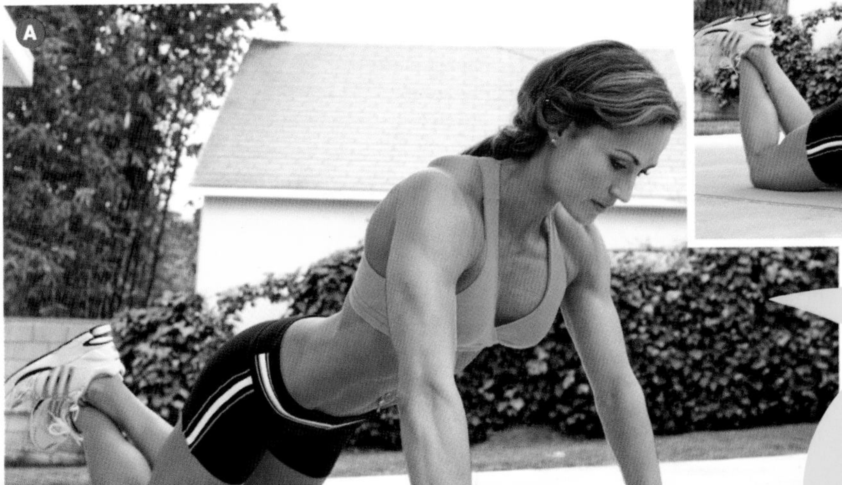
A

**Inside Edge**

***Core stability is the key to good push-up form. If torso stabilization is a challenge, use balance tools as part of your abs training.***

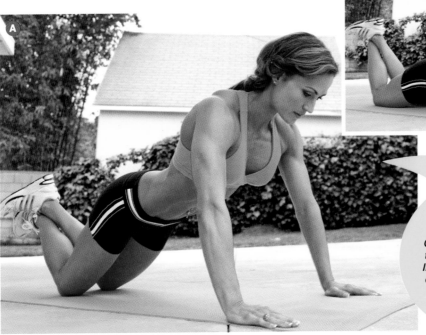

# Machine Chest Press BEGINNER

***Muscles Worked:*** *pectoralis major, anterior deltoid, triceps*

## Technique

1. Sit on a seat that has been adjusted so horizontal handles line up with middle of chest. If handles are modifiable forward or back, adjust so they are several inches in front of chest.
2. Place feet hip-width apart on floor, knees over ankles. Grasp handles, arms straight not locked, wrists neutral.
3. Contract abdominal muscles so spine is neutral; squeeze shoulder blades together and down to stabilize upper back.
4. Maintaining position, bend elbows back so the arms form 90-degree angles, and elbows align with shoulders.
5. Contract chest and triceps muscles to straighten arms, pressing handles away from chest without locking elbows.
6. Pause, then slowly bend elbows to start position.

## Trainer's tips

- Sometimes it's easy to let your arms take over and push. You'll get the most out of this exercise by focusing your effort on the pecs rather than the triceps.
- Check out the new equipment in your gym. A chest press with converging arms, if available, will allow you to press outward while also bringing handles in toward center, allowing you to achieve a fuller contraction.
- To keep pecs firing through the full range of motion, keep shoulders pulled back, especially as you extend the arms.
- For more of a challenge, do a tri-set that includes the machine press with the pec-deck flye and cable crossovers for more intensity.

**Inside Edge**

*The best advantage you can give yourself with this exercise is proper alignment. Take time to adjust the seat and bar to ensure effectiveness.*

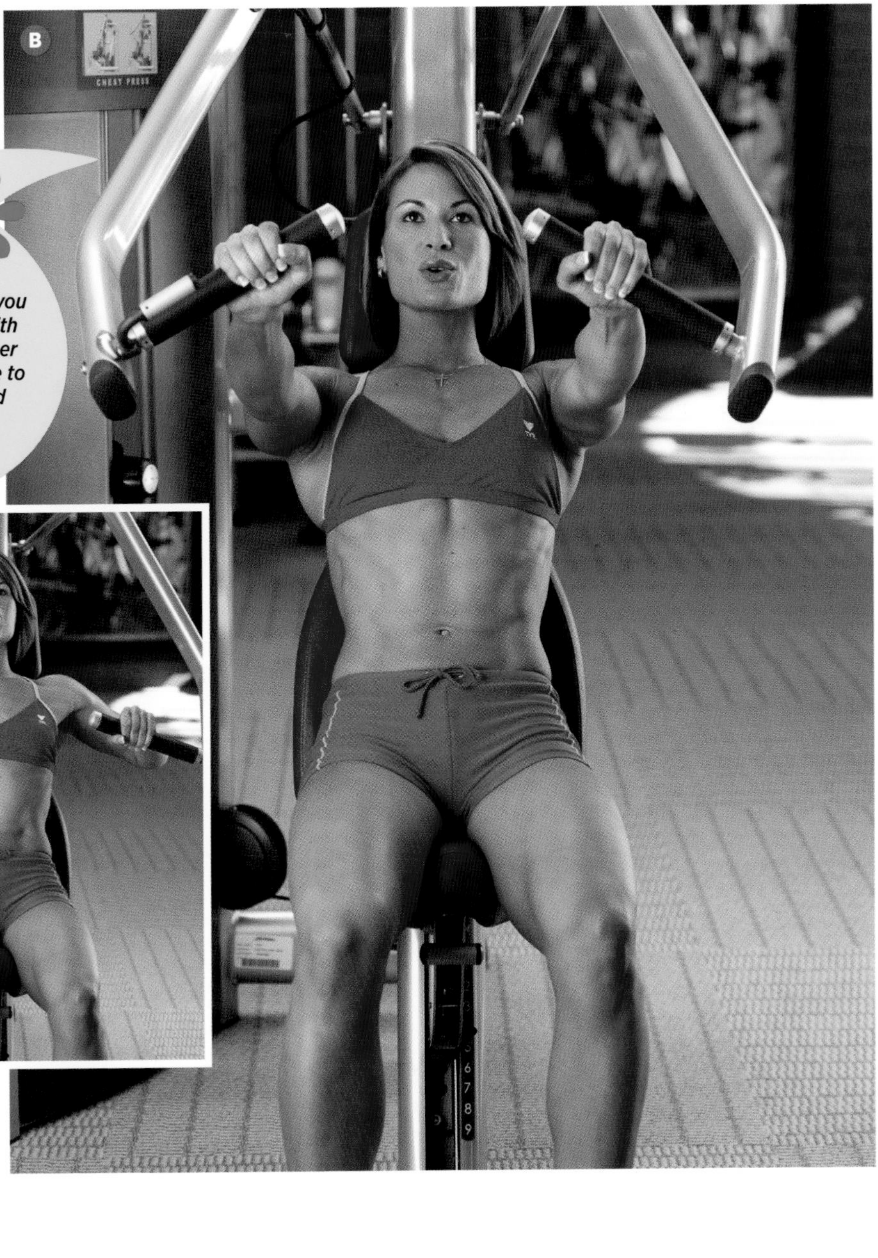


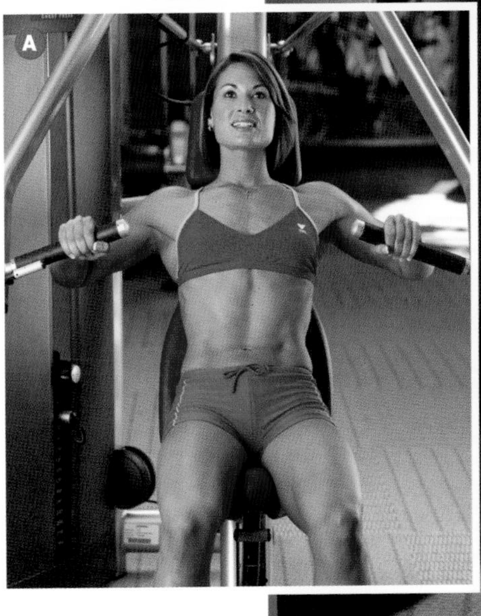

# Standing Cable Flye

INTERMEDIATE/ADVANCED

***Muscles Worked:*** *pectoralis major, anterior deltoid*

## Technique

1. Attach a single cable handle to each upper-cable attachment. Grasp one in each hand in an overhand grip and stand in the middle of the cable cage in a staggered stance.
2. Contract abdominal muscles so your back is in a neutral position, and squeeze shoulder blades together and down.
3. Extend arms out to the sides of your torso at shoulder height and in line with cables, elbows lifted and bent in a soft arc, palms facing in, wrists neutral.
4. Maintaining elbow arc, press handles together in front of you at mid- to lower-chest height until your hands touch.
5. Without rocking, open arms to start position.

## Trainer's tips

- Depending on the height of the cables, you may need to experiment with your torso angle. A higher attachment will dictate a little more forward lean of torso while a lower one will allow for a more upright torso. Adjust accordingly for efficiency.
- Experiment with stance: You may feel more comfortable with feet together or with one leg forward. Your stance should help you feel more stable so you can focus on using your pecs.
- For more of a challenge, do this exercise one arm at a time, keeping the other arm open at chest height. You can also try using the lower cables with an incline bench.

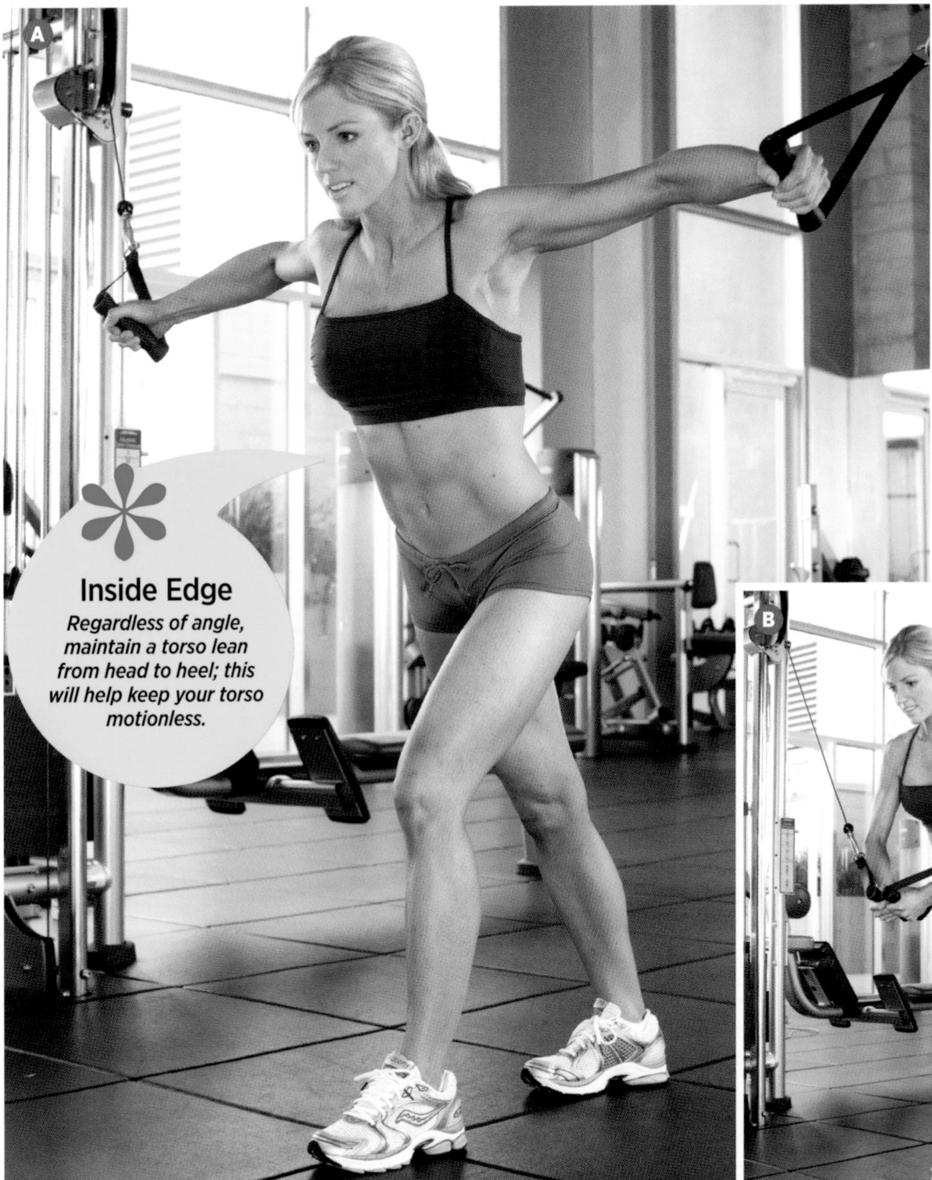


**Inside Edge**

*Regardless of angle, maintain a torso lean from head to heel; this will help keep your torso motionless.*

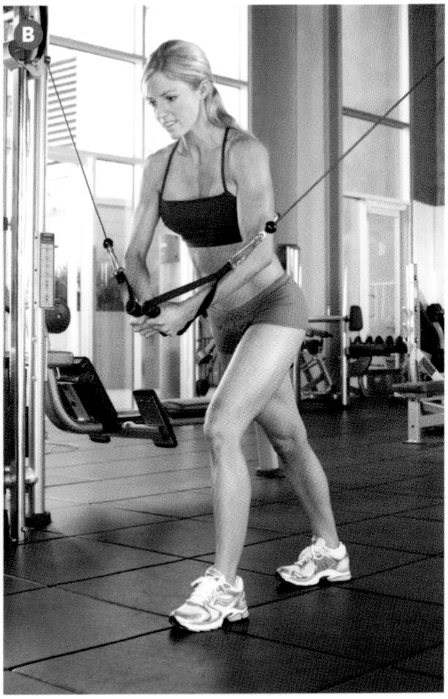

## Beginner Workouts

***Directions:*** ***This is a progressive, six-week program using moderate weight. Do the listed exercises twice a week.***

| WEEK | EXERCISE | SETS | REPS |
|---|---|---|---|
| 1 & 2 | Machine Chest Press | 1–2 | 10–12 |
| | Knee Push-Up | 2 | 8–10 |
| 3 & 4 | Knee Push-Up | 2 | 10–12 |
| | Incline Dumbbell Press | 1–2 | 10–12 |
| 5 & 6 | Ball Push-Up on Thighs | 2 | 8–10 |
| | Flat-Bench Dumbbell Press | 1–2 | 10–12 |
| | Flat-Bench Dumbbell Flye | 1–2 | 10–15 |

**Notes**

*Rest 45–60 seconds between sets. At the end of 6 weeks, progress to intermediate workouts if you're ready.*

## Intermediate Workouts

***Directions:*** ***This is a progressive, six-week program using moderate weight. Do the listed exercises twice a week. If you're using lighter or heavier weight, adjust the number of reps.***

| WEEK | EXERCISE | SETS | REPS |
|---|---|---|---|
| 1 & 2 | Ball Push-Up on Shins | 2 | 8-12 |
| | Incline Dumbbell Press | *1st | 12-15 |
| | **To pyramid sets, increase weight as you decrease reps.* | 2nd | 10-12 |
| | Flat-Bench Dumbbell Flye | 2-3 | 12-15 |
| 3 & 4 | Barbell Bench Press | 1st | 10-12 |
| | Flat-Bench Dumbbell Flye | 2-3 | 10-15 |
| | Incline Dumbbell Press | 2-3 | 10-15 |
| | Ball Push-up on Shins | 2 | 10-12 |
| 5 & 6 | Incline Dumbbell Press | *1st | 12-15 |
| | **To pyramid sets, increase weight as you decrease reps.* | 2nd | 10-12 |
| | Dumbbell Flye (use an incline bench) | 2 | 10-12 |
| | ***Superset:*** | 2 | |
| | Barbell or Dumbbell Press | | 10-12 |
| | Push-Up (ball on shins or full) | | 10-12 |
| | Standing Cable Flye | 2 | 12-15 |

**Notes**

*Rest 60–90 seconds between sets. After six weeks, progress to advanced workouts if you're ready.*

# Advanced Workouts

***Directions:*** ***Perform two workouts a week, choosing from the following programs. You can also do triceps work on the same day or include it as part of a superset program. Adjust reps for lighter or heavier weight.***

| EXERCISE | SETS | REPS |
|---|---|---|
| *Workout 1* | | |
| Incline Dumbbell Press | *1st | 12–15 |
| *To pyramid sets, increase weight as you decrease reps.* | 2 | 8–12 |
| Flat-Bench Dumbbell Flye | 3 | 12–15 |
| ***Superset:*** | 3 | |
| Barbell Bench Press | | 10–12 |
| Full Push-Up | | 10–15 |
| Incline Low-Cable Flye | 3 | 12–15 |
| *Workout 2* | | |
| Standing Cable Flye | 3 | 10–12 |
| Flat-Bench Dumbbell Press | 3 | 12–15 |
| ***Superset:*** | 3 | |
| Ball Push-Up on Shins | | 12–15 |
| Dumbbell Flye (use ball instead of bench) | | 10–12 |
| Incline Dumbbell Press | 3 | 10–15 |
| *Workout 3* | | |
| Full Push-Up | 3 | 10–15 |
| Incline Low-Cable Flye | 3 | 10–12 |
| ***Superset :*** | 3 | |
| Barbell Bench Press | | 8–12 |
| Flat-Bench Dumbbell Flye | | 10–12 |

***Notes***

*Rest 60–90 seconds between sets.*

# Can't-Get-to-the-Gym Workouts

***Directions:*** ***Do the following exercises when you want to work out at home or on the road. Change the order for variety. For superset work, add triceps exercises.***

| EXERCISE | SETS | REPS |
|---|---|---|
| Push-Up (knee*, full or ball version) | 2–3 | 10–15 |
| Dumbbell Press (either with a bench* or rolled towel under shoulders) | 2–3 | 8–15 |
| Flat-Bench Dumbbell Flye* | 2–3 | 10–15 |

***Notes***

*Rest 60–90 seconds between sets. If you're a beginner, only do the exercises marked with an asterisk (*).*

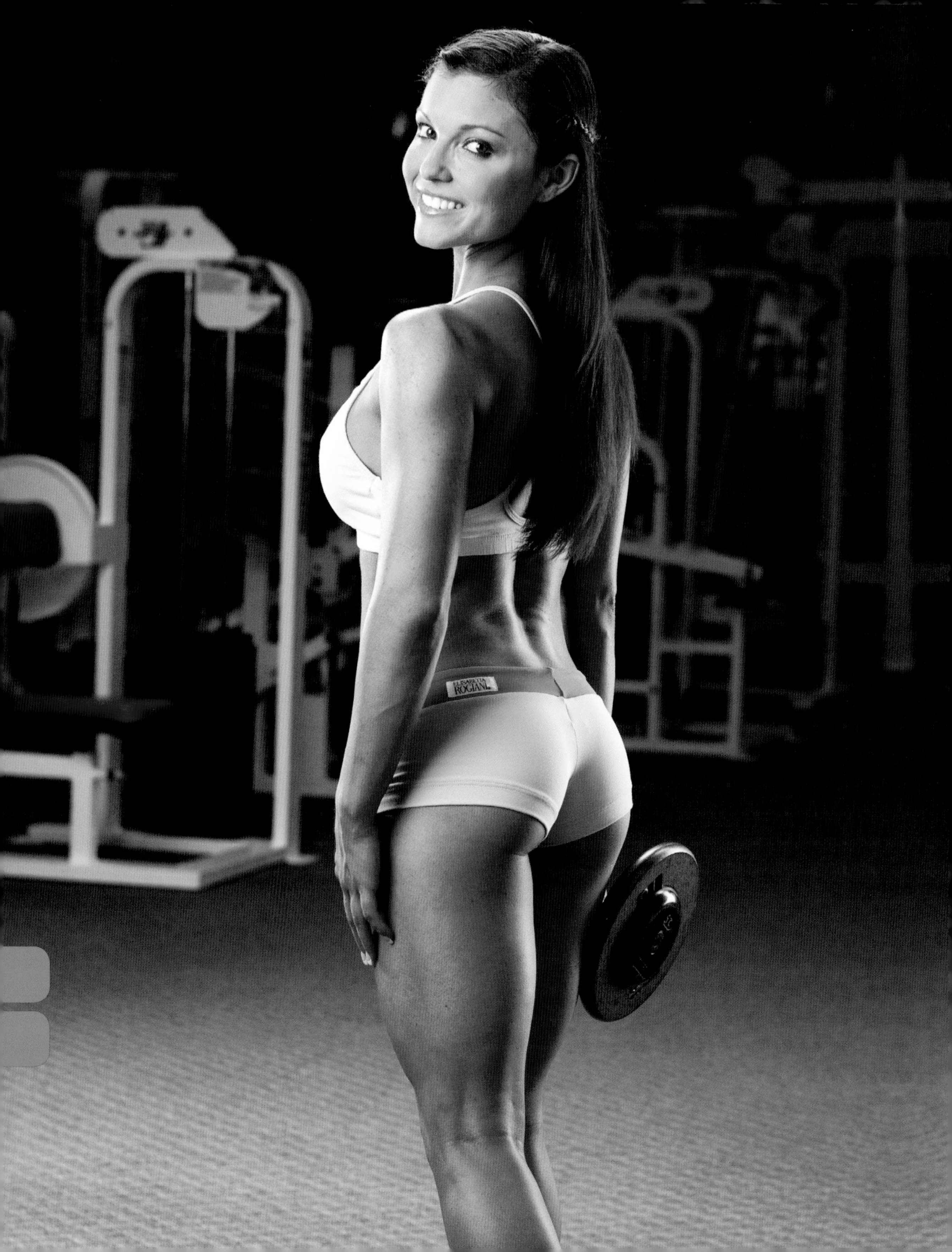

Chapter 7

# Glutes & Legs

*Solutions to firm up your entire lower body.*

THE GLUTEUS MAXIMUS is the largest and most superficial of the gluteal muscles. The maximus originates on the outer edge of your pelvis and attaches to the rear thighbone. The gluteus maximus is responsible for hip extension, which lifts your leg behind you and rotates your thighbone outward. Hip abductors are the gluteal muscles that form your upper hips. The primary hip abductor, the gluteus medius, attaches to your pelvis and top of your thighbone. It moves your leg out and away from your body's midline with the help of the gluteus minimus, which is located underneath it, and four other assistor muscles. The opposite gluteus medius also works to keep your pelvis from tilting when standing on one leg.

The three hamstring muscles (biceps femoris, semimembranosus, semitendinosus) attach to the "sit bones" at the base of your butt and run lengthwise along the underside of your thigh to attach just below the knee on your lower leg bones. They work with the gluteus maximus during hip extension and are independently responsible for flexing your knees. Both of these muscle groups also work with the quadriceps and hip abductors and adductors for multi-muscle exercises. The hip and thigh muscles work together with the gluteals and calves during multi-muscle exercises. Any of these muscles can also be isolated.

Your thigh muscles are comprised of the four quadriceps muscles on the front of each thigh which flex the hip and extend the knee; the three hamstring muscles on the rear of the thighs which extend the hip and flex the knee; and adductor muscles which form your inner thighs and work to bring your leg toward your body's midline. Five primary muscles run along your inner thigh, connecting to your pubic bone and thighbone: the three muscles of the adductor group (longus, brevis and magnus) and the pectineus and gracilis; the latter two also flex your hip. In particular, the abductors (upper hip) and adductors primarily work with the quadriceps to stabilize your legs to ensure proper alignment and protect your knees. The iliopsoas (hip flexors) are also involved, and activate when you bend at the hips.

# Alternating Reverse Bench Lunge

INTERMEDIATE/ADVANCED

***Muscles Worked:*** *gluteus maximus, quadriceps, hamstrings, calves; gluteus medius and hip adductors as stabilizers*

## Technique

1. Holding a dumbbell in each hand, arms hanging at sides, palms facing in, stand on top of a weight bench or an 8- to 12-inch step. Feet are hip-width apart, legs straight but not locked.
2. Contract abdominal muscles so spine is in neutral position. Squeeze shoulder blades together and down to stabilize your upper back.
3. Without leaning torso, step back and down to floor with one foot, bending both knees so front knee aligns over ankle, back knee points toward floor and back heel is lifted.
4. Push off foot on floor, using glutes and thigh muscles to straighten both legs and return to start position. Alternate legs to equal one rep.

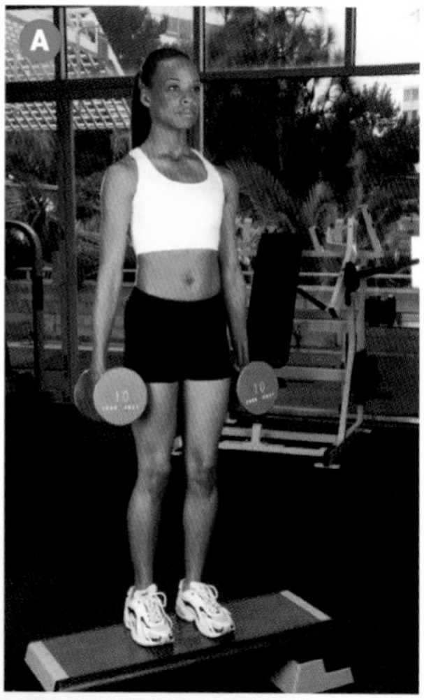


## Trainer's tips

- Avoid ankle and foot strain by paying attention to how you step down. Touch first with the toes, gently rolling through the foot and softly bending the knee as heel stays lifted. Reverse as you step back up, pushing off the ball of foot and then the toes. Use the foot and ankle as natural shock absorbers.
- Allowing dumbbells to swing as you step down and back up will make it harder to keep torso erect and stable. Use back and shoulder muscles to keep your arms stationary.
- For a killer workout, superset this exercise with walking lunges and Smith-machine lunges. Finish with a set of unweighted jump squats.

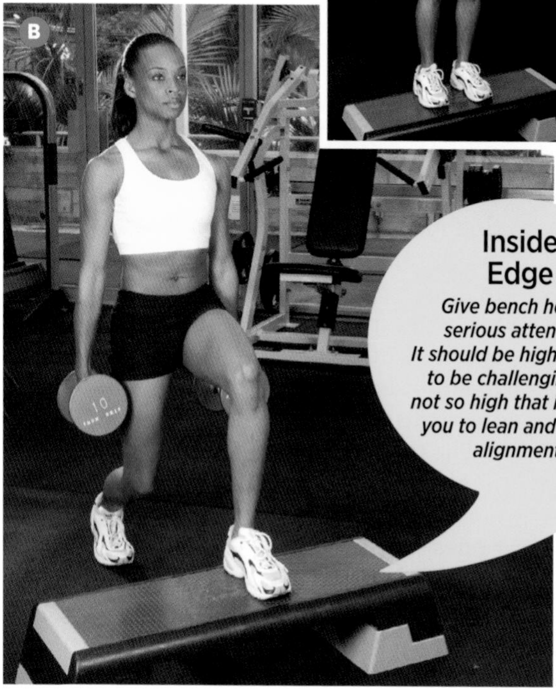


**Inside Edge**

*Give bench height serious attention: It should be high enough to be challenging but not so high that it causes you to lean and distort alignment.*

# Ball Bridge

INTERMEDIATE/ADVANCED

***Muscles Worked:*** *gluteus maximus, upper fibers of hamstrings; erector spinae and abdominals as stabilizers*

## Technique

1. Lying faceup on the floor, arms relaxed by your sides and palms down, place both heels on top of a medicine ball with knees bent about 90 degrees.
2. Contract abdominal muscles so your spine is in a neutral position. Squeeze shoulder blades together and down to stabilize upper back against the floor.
3. Contract glutes and press heels down against the ball to slowly lift hips off the floor until you're supporting your body weight on upper back and heels. Your body forms a straight line from shoulders to knees.
4. Hold for two counts, then slowly lower hips to floor.

## Trainer's tips

- As you lift, focus on the glutes by contracting throughout the entire range of motion.
- Keep hands loose; don't press them into the floor and try not to take tension into the upper back and shoulders as you lift.
- It's important to lift hips, but lifting them too high will cause back strain.
- If the ball is too challenging, practice the lifting motion by placing heels on a bench, then switch to the ball when you're ready.
- This exercise is a great complement to deadlifts and cable kickbacks. For more intensity, superset all three exercises.
- For more of a challenge, perform this exercise with one leg at a time.

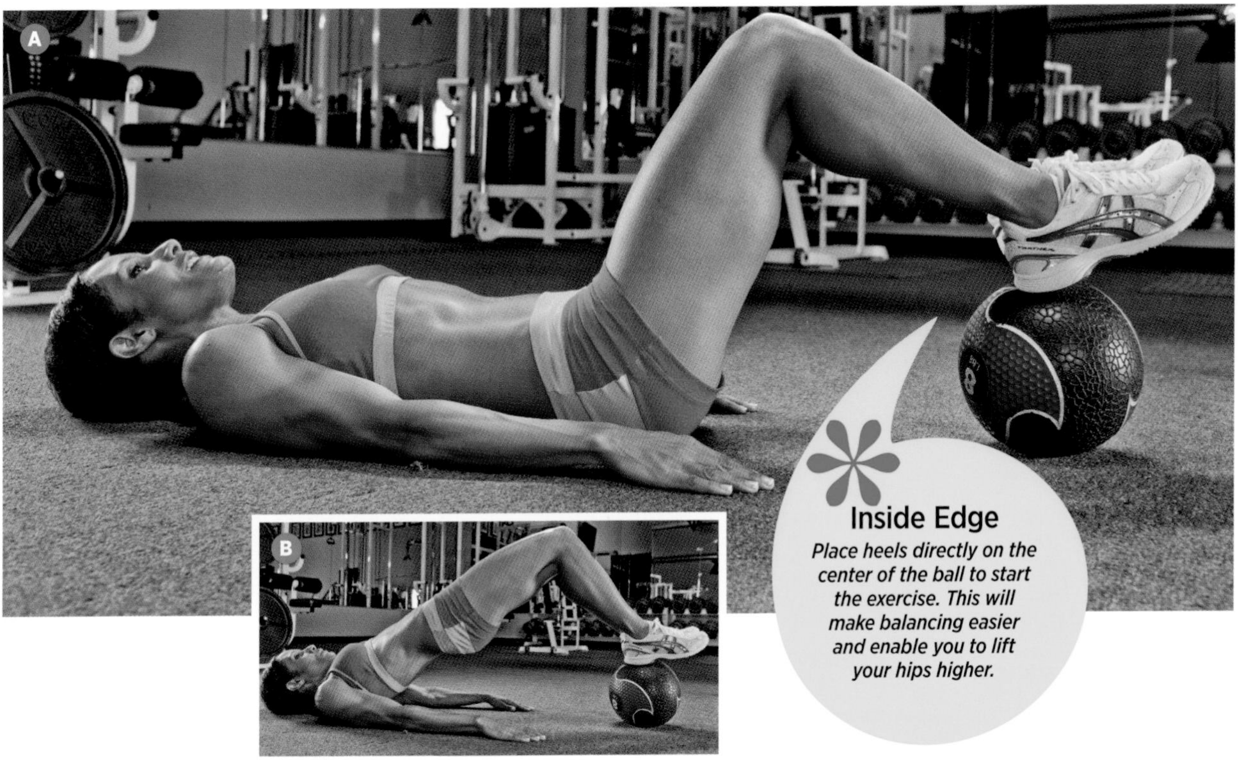


**Inside Edge**

*Place heels directly on the center of the ball to start the exercise. This will make balancing easier and enable you to lift your hips higher.*

# Ball Bridge Curl INTERMEDIATE/ADVANCED

***Muscles Worked:*** *hamstrings, with emphasis on lower fibers; gluteus maximus, erector spinae and abdominals as stabilizers*

## Technique

1. Lie faceup on floor, arms relaxed at sides, palms facing down. Place ankles on top of a stability ball; keep legs straight.
2. Contract abdominal muscles so spine is in neutral position, and squeeze shoulder blades together and down.
3. Contract glutes, pressing heels into ball to lift hips off floor so your upper back, head and arms are in contact with floor, your body forming one straight line from shoulders to heels.
4. Maintain lifted position and bend knees, pulling ball toward hips with heels until thighs are vertical.
5. Pause at the top, then roll ball back out by pushing it away with heels until legs are straight, keeping hips raised in bridge position.

## Trainer's tips

- Don't let hips drop; this takes part of the load off the glutes and reduces your range of motion.
- As you contract the hamstrings, make sure the ball is rolling toward you in a straight line. Put even pressure on the ball with both heels and pull evenly with both hamstrings.
- In the bridge position, shift weight onto your shoulders and upper back, not your neck.
- For more control, begin the exercise with calves (instead of ankles) on the ball.
- For more of a challenge, perform this exercise by rolling the ball with one leg at a time.

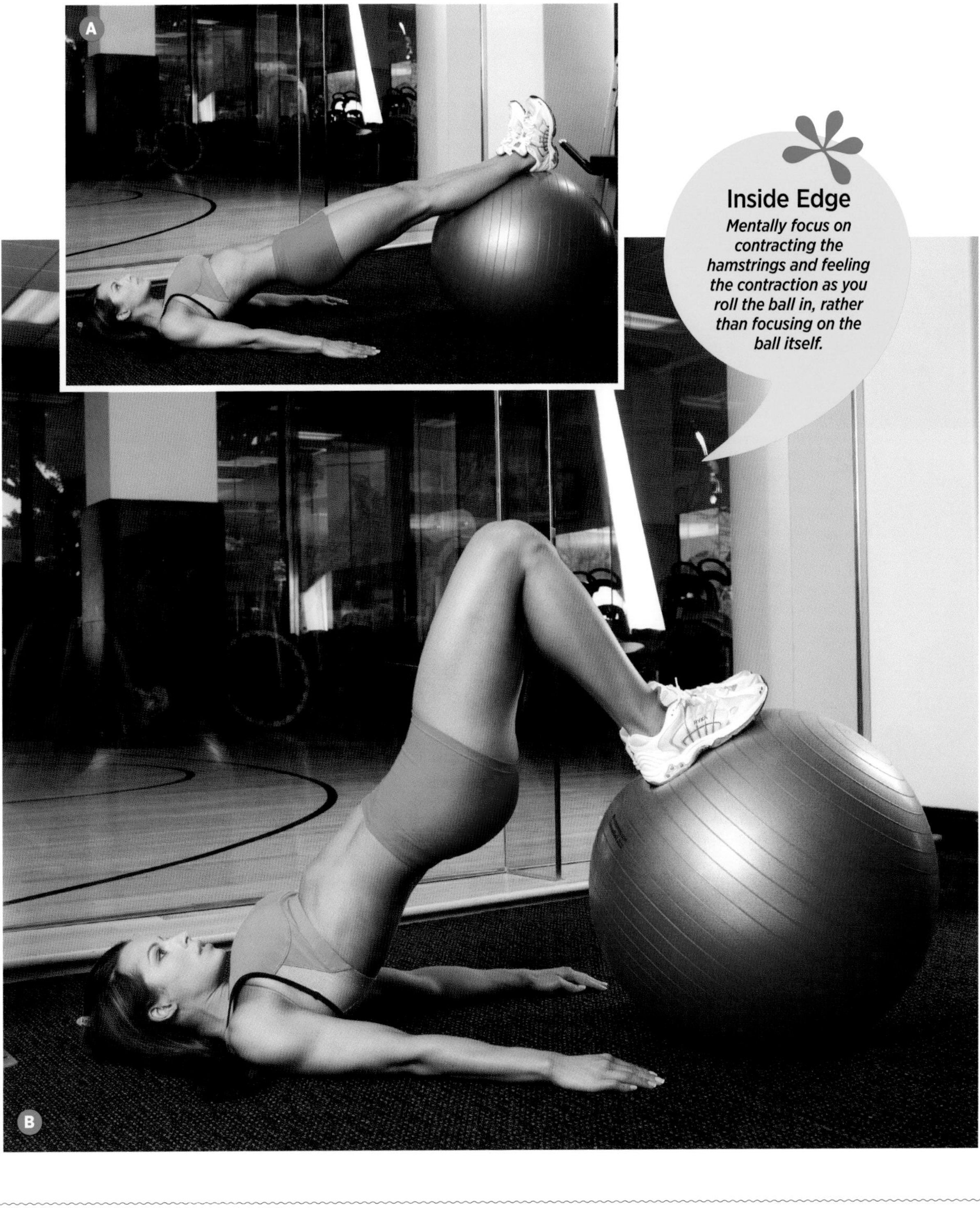


**Inside Edge**

*Mentally focus on contracting the hamstrings and feeling the contraction as you roll the ball in, rather than focusing on the ball itself.*

# Ball Glute Lift

BEGINNER/INTERMEDIATE

***Muscles Worked:*** *gluteus maximus, hip adductors, hamstrings; abdominals and spine extensors as stabilizers*

**Inside Edge**

***Continue to draw tailbone down as you raise your legs; this will minimize balance problems and enable you to maximize the glutes contraction.***

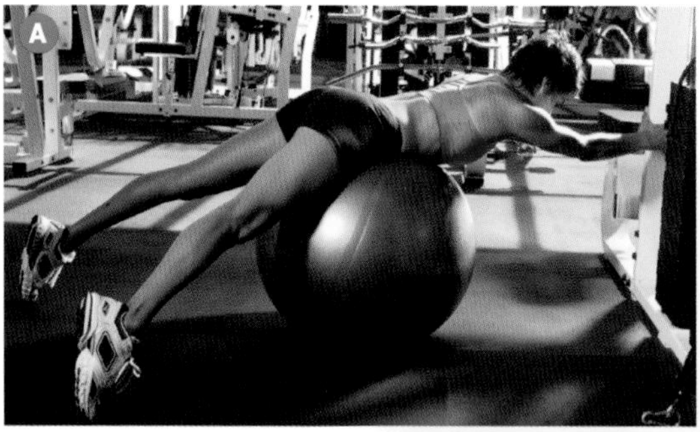


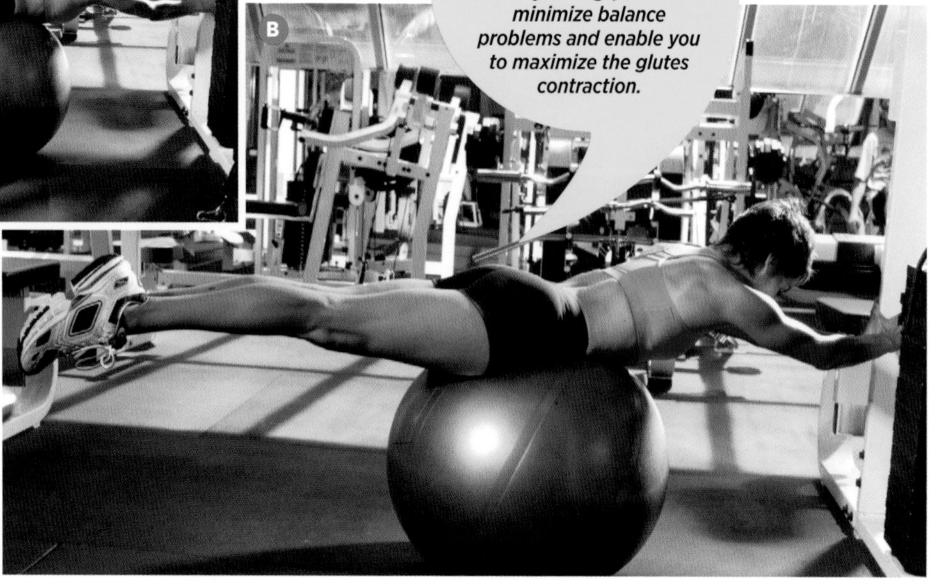


## Technique

1. Drape yourself facedown over a stability ball so you're lying on the ball and supported from lower rib cage to hips.
2. Holding a support in front of you with both hands, extend legs, separating them wider than hip-width apart in a V, toes touching the floor.
3. Contract your abdominal muscles, dropping tailbone down so torso forms a straight line from head to hips. Squeeze shoulder blades together and down to stabilize your upper back.
4. Tighten glutes, slowly raising legs up to hip height. Use inner thighs to bring legs together at the top of the movement.
5. Pause, then slowly lower legs to start position.

## Trainer's tips

- Keep torso motionless by maintaining abdominal contraction so the glutes do all the work. Imagine your abs as a corset, wrapping all the way around your torso; the more stable you are the better your balance and the sooner you'll be able to add resistance.
- Don't swing your legs up and use momentum; keep consistent tension on your glutes and keep legs straight.
- For variety, adjust your position so the front of your hips are just off the ball; this maximizes hip extension and the amount of work your glutes do.
- Keep shoulders down and relaxed, head and neck aligned with spine.
- For more of a challenge, add resistance with ankle weights.

# Ball Wall Squat BEGINNER

***Muscles Worked:*** *gluteus maximus, quadriceps, hamstrings; hip abductors and adductors as stabilizers*

## Technique

1. Place a stability ball between a wall and the small of your back. Holding a dumbbell in each hand, arms hanging by your sides, palms in, walk both feet forward 1–2 feet. The ball supports your torso.
2. Contract abdominal muscles so spine is in a neutral position, and squeeze shoulder blades together and down to stabilize upper back.
3. Keeping torso vertical, bend knees and lower hips toward floor until thighs are approximately parallel to the floor and knees are bent at 90 degrees; don't let hips press back as you lower.
4. Using glutes and thigh muscles, straighten legs to start position without locking knees.

### Inside Edge

***Keeping tailbone pointing toward floor emphasizes the glutes. To involve the quads more, allow hips to move slightly backward at the bottom of the squat.***

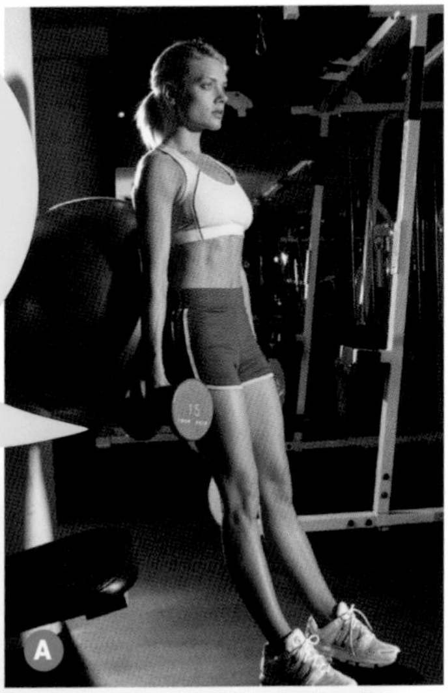

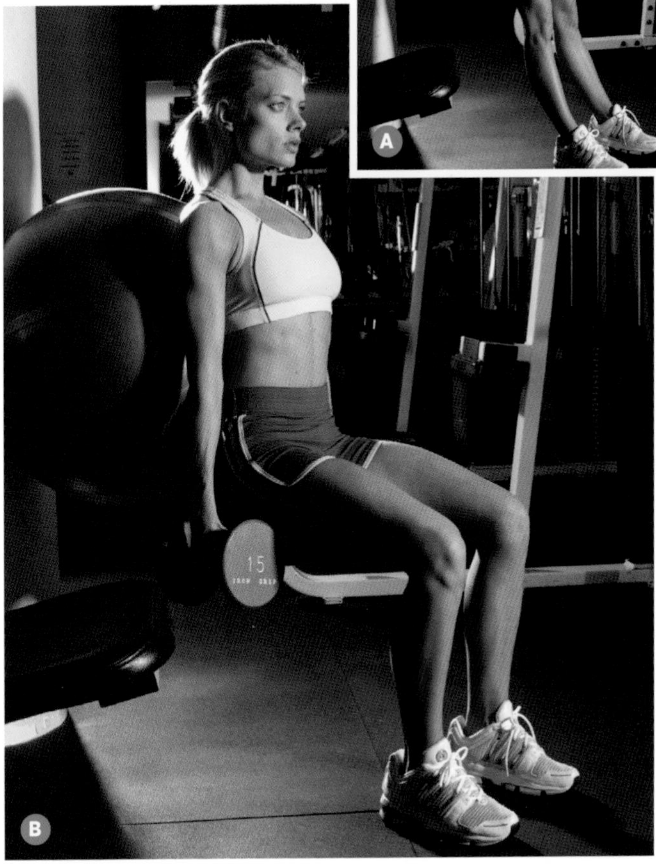

## Trainer's tips

- Walk feet far enough forward to keep knees aligned with ankles in the lower position; your entire body will be at a slight lean when you start.
- The support of the ball allows you to squat deeper than if you were freestanding and also allows you to use heavier weights.
- Reap greater benefit in the glutes by pushing with the heels as you drive your hips up and out of the squat.
- For even more glutes emphasis, pause for a count of three at the bottom, then tighten glutes before you straighten legs.
- For more of a challenge, lift one foot off the floor and perform as a one-legged squat.

# Cable Kickback INTERMEDIATE/ADVANCED

***Muscles Worked:** gluteus maximus, upper fibers of hamstrings*

## Technique

1. Attach an ankle cuff to a low-cable pulley and right ankle, then stand facing weight stack, left foot on a 10-pound weight plate or other raised surface, knee slightly bent and one hand on support bar. Hold right foot a few inches off floor and in front of torso, leg straight but not locked, foot slightly flexed.
2. Contract abdominal muscles so spine is in a neutral position, and squeeze shoulder blades together and down to stabilize upper back.
3. Keeping knee straight, torso erect, shoulders and hips square, lead with heel as you use glutes to lift right leg behind you.
4. Hold for two counts, then lower leg, leading with toes.
5. Repeat for reps, then switch legs.

## Trainer's tips

- Avoid arching your back as you lift the leg; this won't add to the glutes' workload and will place strain on the lower back.
- If you experience back discomfort, kneel with supporting leg on an incline bench placed lengthwise in front of the stack. Allow torso to lean forward on seat back while performing reps, which also eliminates the temptation to cheat with torso.
- To activate upper gluteus maximus fibers, rotate the working leg out from the hips, toes pointing up at the end of the movement.
- For a quick superset, perform standing cable abduction, cable adduction and cable kickbacks on the same leg back-to-back. Switch legs and then finish with walking lunges.

B

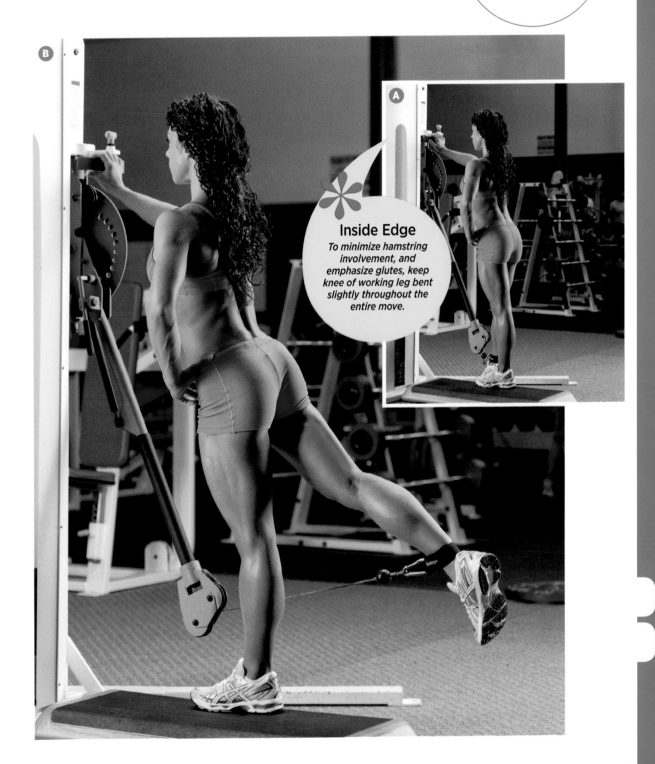

A

**Inside Edge**

*To minimize hamstring involvement, and emphasize glutes, keep knee of working leg bent slightly throughout the entire move.*

# Jump Squat INTERMEDIATE/ADVANCED

***Muscles Worked:*** *gluteus maximus, quadriceps, hamstrings, calves; hip abductors and adductors as stabilizers*

## Technique

1. Stand with feet hip-width apart, legs straight but not locked, toes pointing forward. Bend elbows loosely by your sides and hold forearms in front of you, hands relaxed.
2. Contract abdominal muscles so spine is in a neutral position, and squeeze shoulder blades together and down.
3. Bend knees, lowering hips back and down toward floor until knee bend approaches 90 degrees and they are aligned over ankles. Chest remains lifted as you swing arms back.
4. Using glutes, thighs and calf muscles, forcefully drive hips back up through start position, straightening legs until feet leave the floor in a jump, arms reaching overhead.
5. As you return to floor, gently roll through the feet, bending knees and bringing arms back into the next squat.

## Trainer's tips

- Check your alignment at the bottom of the squat: Make sure knees haven't drifted inward which makes the jump less effective and can lead to knee injury.
- Choose a softer surface with more "give." Most free-weight areas use high-density rubber flooring that will reduce the jarring upon landing.
- Increase the height of your jump by thrusting your arms up as you jump and reaching them behind you as you land.
- To increase difficulty, hold a medicine ball close to your chest as you jump.

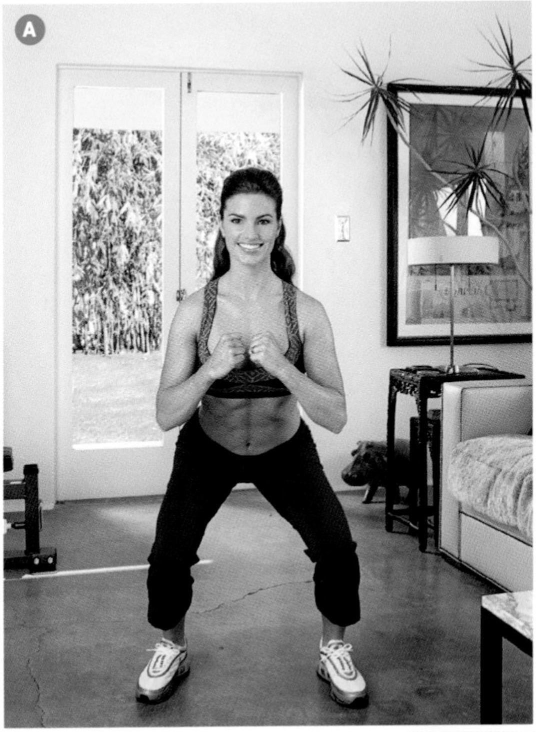


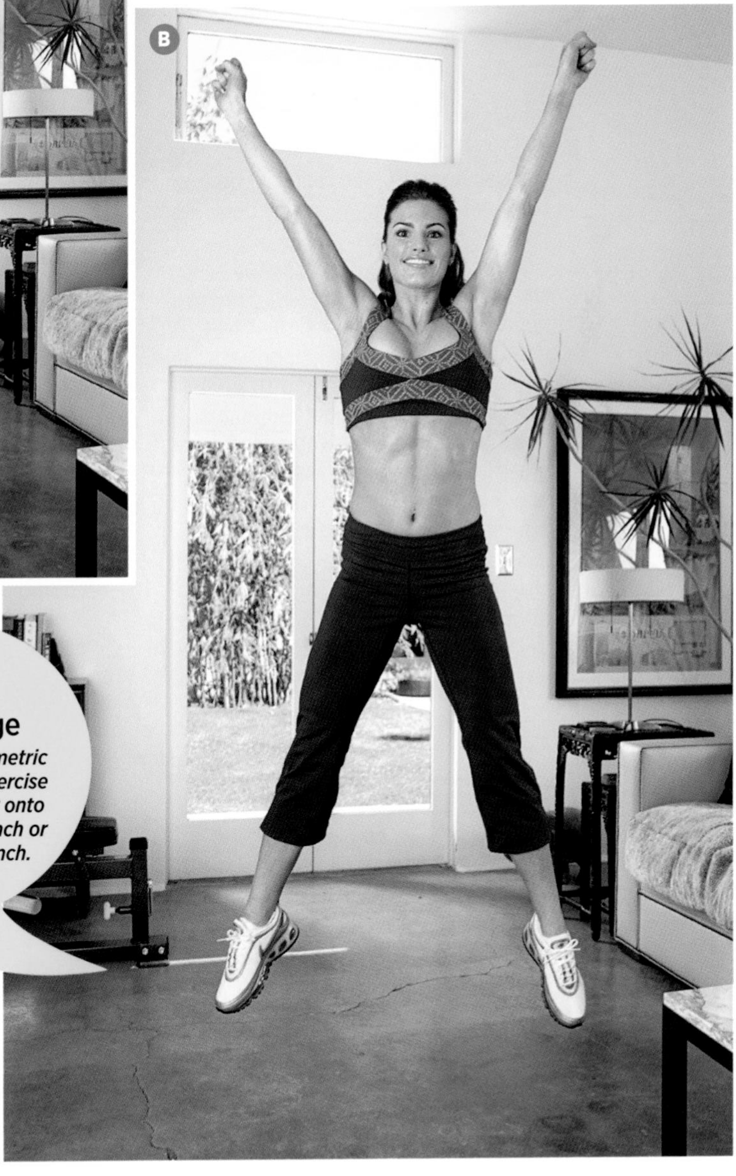


**Inside Edge**

*Increase the plyometric benefits of this exercise by jumping either onto or from a step bench or short weight bench.*

# Leg Press **BEGINNER/INTERMEDIATE/ADVANCED**

***Muscles Worked:*** *gluteus maximus, quadriceps, hamstrings; hip abductors and adductors as stabilizers*

## Technique

1. Adjust a leg press to 45 degrees then sit, placing both feet centered on foot plate, hip-width apart, knees bent. Hold handles for support.
2. Contract abdominal muscles so your spine is in a neutral position. Squeeze your shoulder blades together and down to stabilize your upper back. Release machine locks and straighten legs, keeping knees and feet aligned.
3. Bend knees, slowly lowering the plate in a controlled manner, keeping knees aligned with ankles, until your thighs approach vertical or you lose neutral lower spine position.
4. Using your glutes and thigh muscles, straighten legs by pressing plate away until knees are straight but not locked.

## Trainer's tips

- To protect your lower back, make sure you maintain a neutral lower back curve throughout the rep; going too heavy and bending knees too deep can cause back to arch.
- Focus on keeping chest lifted and shoulders down as you press away.
- Experiment with stance. Placing feet a little higher on the plate will emphasize hamstrings and glutes; a lower stance will more greatly target quads. Try a wide, turned-out stance to activate inner thighs.
- To increase the intensity, work with a partner so you can do drop sets: Load press with several smaller plates and have a partner strip them away one at a time on your last set.

## Inside Edge

*Poor knee alignment affects form and your ability to train with heavy weight. Track knees with center of feet so they don't roll in or out.*

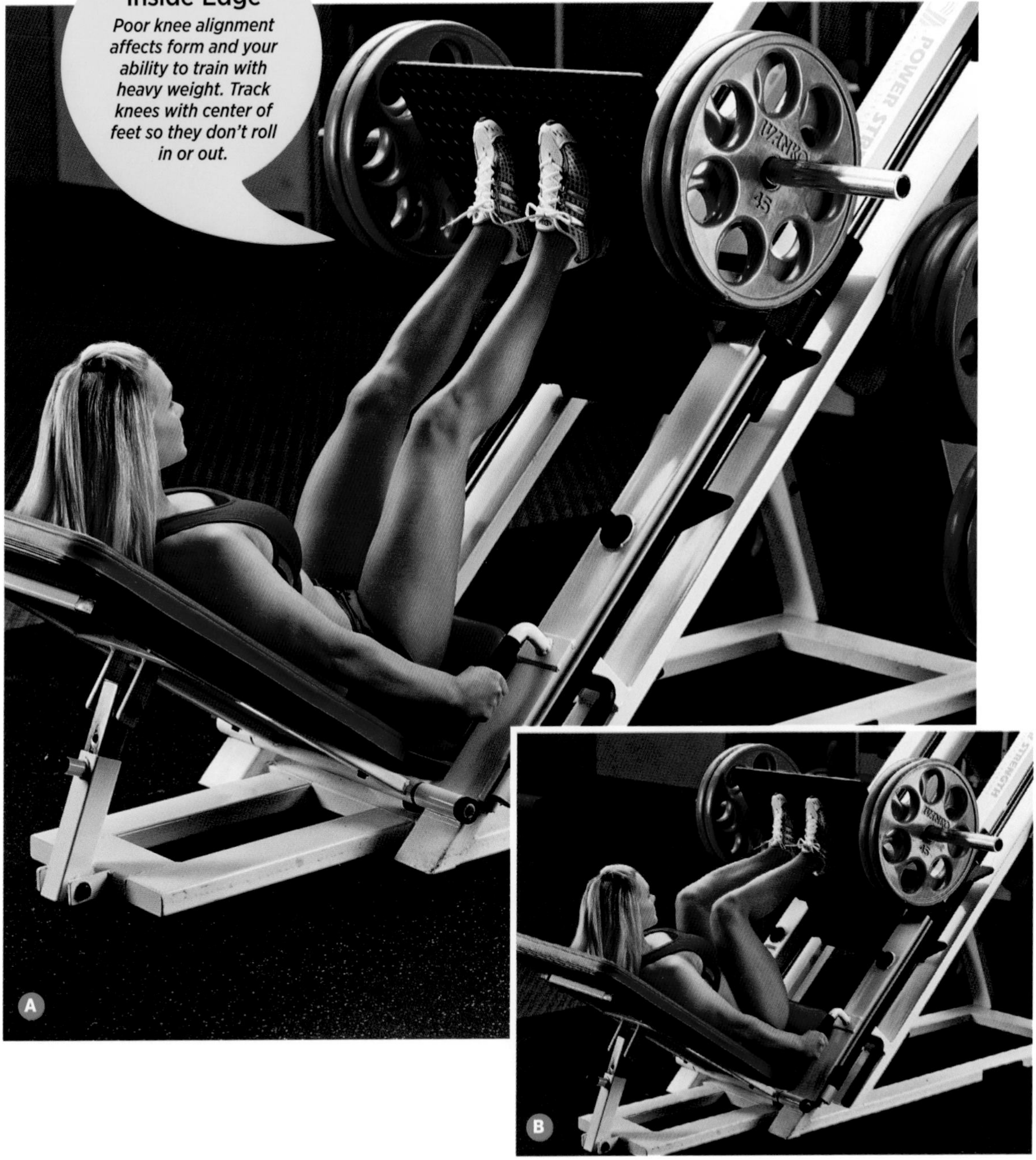

# Plié Dumbbell Squat

BEGINNER/ INTERMEDIATE/ADVANCED

***Muscles Worked:*** *gluteus maximus, quadriceps, hamstrings, hip adductors*

## Technique

1. Standing with feet wider than hip-width apart, legs straight and rotated out comfortably from the hips, hold a single dumbbell vertically with cupped hands underneath top plate. Arms are straight and hang in front of body.
2. Contract abdominal muscles so spine is in a neutral position, tailbone pointing toward floor. Squeeze shoulder blades together and down to stabilize upper back.
3. Bend knees, keeping feet and knees aligned, lowering hips toward floor only as low as you can without tilting pelvis; keep heels down and weight evenly distributed over feet.
4. Focus on squeezing inner thighs together as you straighten legs to start position without locking knees.

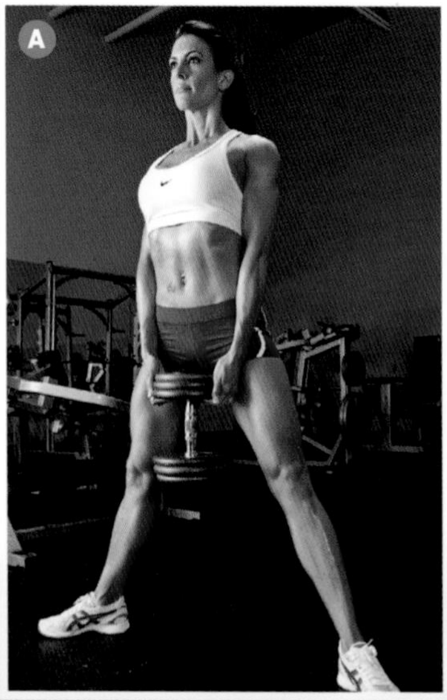

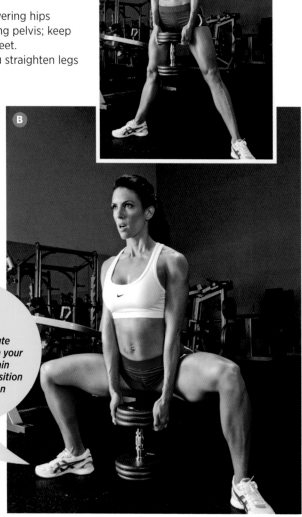
A

## Trainer's tips

- Keep torso vertical, tailbone pointing toward floor when lowering and standing. (Shifting hips backwards turns the plié into a squat.)
- Don't over-rotate feet. Begin the rotation from hips to ensure proper alignment of knees out over feet as you lower. Turning feet out more than hips places a great deal of stress on knee joints.
- For variety, perform with a barbell across upper back and shoulders or use a Smith machine. You can also try standing in the center of a length of tubing, handles held at shoulders.
- For more of a challenge, stand on a balance tool or alternate side squats, stepping out to one side then drawing legs together.

**Inside Edge**

***To encourage glute work, press through your heels and maintain turned-out knee position as you straighten your legs.***

B

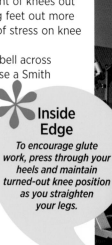

# Reverse/Front Lunge

BEGINNER/ INTERMEDIATE/ADVANCED

***Muscles Worked:*** *gluteus maximus, quadriceps, hamstrings, calves; gluteus medius and hip adductors as stabilizers*

## Technique

1. Holding a dumbbell in each hand, arms hanging down at sides and palms facing in, stand with feet hip-width apart and legs straight but not locked.
2. Contract abdominal muscles so spine is neutral. Squeeze shoulder blades together and down.
3. Take a step back (or forward for front lunges) with one foot, toes pointing forward and other leg extended behind you, heel lifted. Bend knees, lowering hips toward floor until front knee is bent at 90 degrees and back knee is pointing down; back heel remains lifted.
4. Using glutes and thigh muscles, straighten both legs, pressing hips back up to starting position.
5. Either repeat for reps or alternate legs.

### Inside Edge

***Develop a rhythmic cadence to your reps. Add a visual focus and coordinate your breathing with the reps for a meditative-like focus.***

## Trainer's tips

- Include forward and reverse lunges in your workout. Both require different types of body awareness that can complement other exercise pursuits.
- If you've done only stationary lunges in the past, this exercise will take your workouts up a notch.
- As you lunge either forward or backward, keep torso erect and centered between both legs so you don't lean into the lunge.
- Don't let front knee wander inward or past toes; this strains knee tissue.
- Use a barbell for variety, but pay extra attention to keeping torso erect. With weight higher on your torso, the exercise will be more challenging.

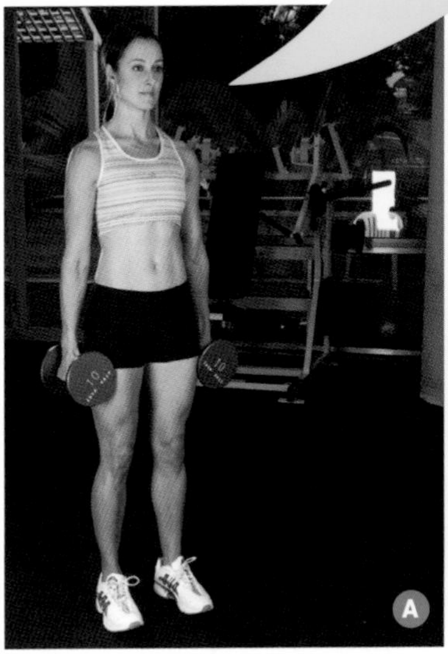
A

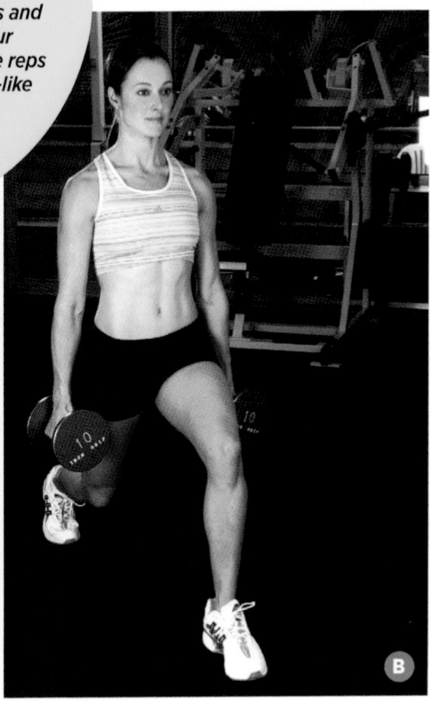
B

# Romanian Deadlift INTERMEDIATE/ADVANCED

***Muscles Worked:*** *gluteus maximus, upper fibers of hamstrings; erector spinae and abdominals as stabilizers*

## Technique

1. Stand with feet hip-width apart, legs straight but not locked. Hold a barbell with an overhand grip about shoulder-width apart, arms straight so bar hangs in front of thighs.
2. Contract abdominal muscles so spine is in a neutral position. Squeeze shoulder blades together and down to stabilize your upper back.
3. Keeping chest lifted and torso straight, bend knees slightly and hinge forward from hips, bar hanging in line with shoulders until you feel a stretch in your hamstrings.
4. Use glutes and hamstrings to straighten torso to an erect standing position, knees still slightly bent.
5. Pause, then hinge forward and repeat for reps.

## Trainer's tips

- Your range of motion depends on your ability to maintain the neutral curve in your lower back. Check lower-back position sideways in a mirror as you hinge forward. If you begin to round your spine, increase your knee bend and bring torso up slightly from parallel.
- As you increase the weight, it will become more challenging to keep your shoulder blades together.
- To strengthen your scapular stabilizers, loop tubing around a support, grasp handles with both hands and squeeze shoulder blades together. Hold for three counts. Repeat 10 times.
- Keep the bar close to your body; otherwise it compensates back muscles and takes efficiency away from glutes and hamstrings.

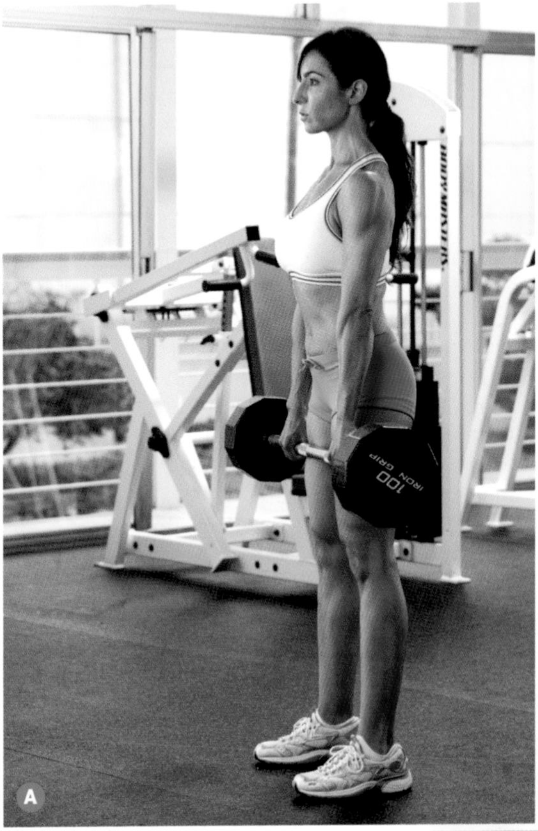


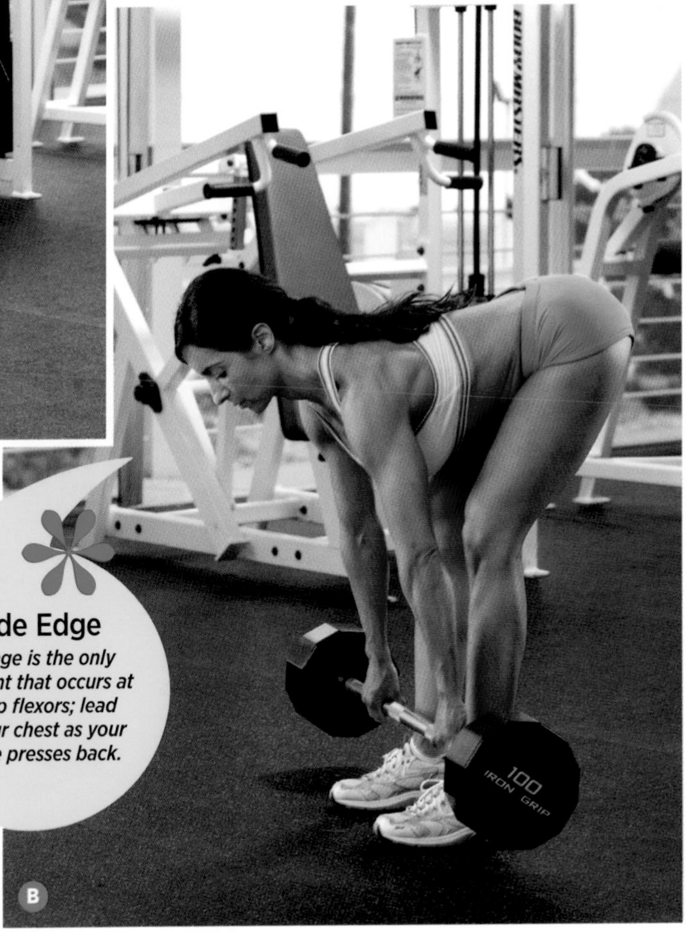


**Inside Edge**

*The hinge is the only movement that occurs at your hip flexors; lead with your chest as your tailbone presses back.*

# Seated Abduction

**BEGINNER/INTERMEDIATE**

***Muscles Worked:*** *gluteus medius, upper fibers of gluteus maximus*

## Technique

1. Sit upright on the seat of a hip abductor machine with your entire back against seat pad. Place your feet flat on footrests with the outsides of your knees against the thigh pads, knees aligned over your ankles.
2. Contract abdominal muscles so spine is in a neutral position, and squeeze shoulder blades together and down to stabilize your upper back.
3. Using your upper-hip muscles, press your knees out and away from the center of your body to a comfortably open position (about hip-width apart). Chest is lifted and abdominals remain tight.
4. Hold for two counts, then slowly return to the start position without knees touching.

## Trainer's tips

- This is a relatively safe exercise to use heavy weights, but pay attention to your form. Don't push your back into the pad to "help" complete a heavier set. Keeping the torso erect and stable causes the upper hips to work harder.
- Don't bounce at the end of the range of motion, which uses momentum instead of muscular effort and can injure the groin area.
- For a change of pace, use a multi-hip machine or attach an ankle collar and perform the exercise standing with a low cable.
- For more intensity, do a set of dumbbell side lunges followed by a drop set of seated abduction, then repeat for desired sets.

**Inside Edge**

***For an intense upper-hip workout, imagine your thighs as the hands of a clock slowly moving from 12 to 10 and 2.***

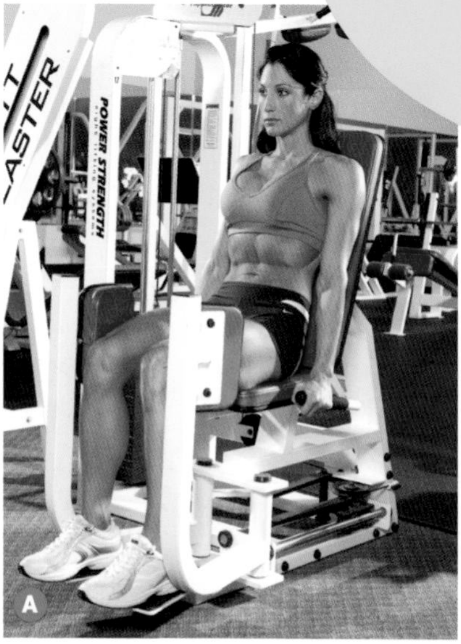


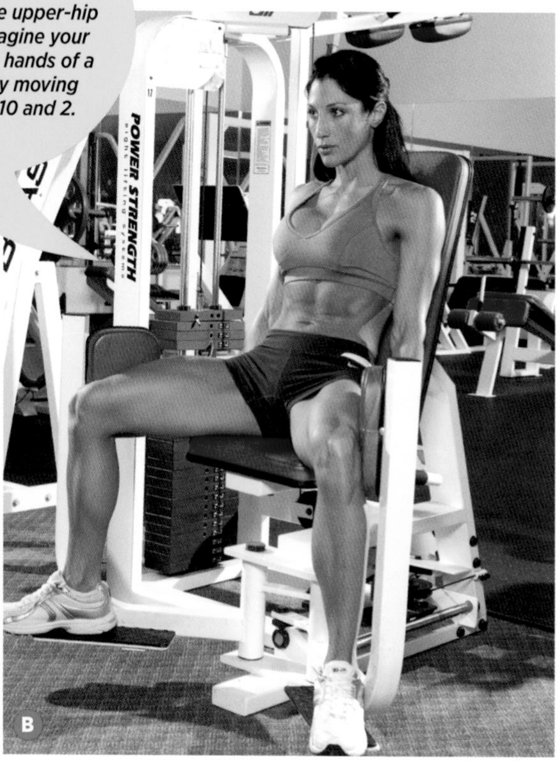

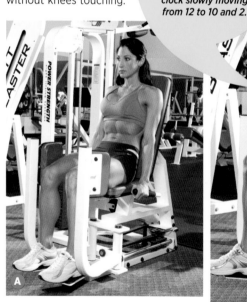

# Seated Adduction

BEGINNER/INTERMEDIATE

***Muscles worked:** hip adductors*

## Technique

1. Sit upright on a hip adductor machine with your back in full contact with the back pad. Adjust the leg levers so legs are open to a comfortable position, no more than hip-width apart, and place feet on the footrests with insides of knees against the thigh pads, knees aligned over ankles.
2. Contract abdominal muscles so spine is in a neutral position. Squeeze shoulder blades together and down to stabilize your upper back.
3. Using inner-thigh muscles, press leg pads in toward the midline of your body without allowing pads to touch in the center.
4. Hold for two counts, then slowly open legs to start position.

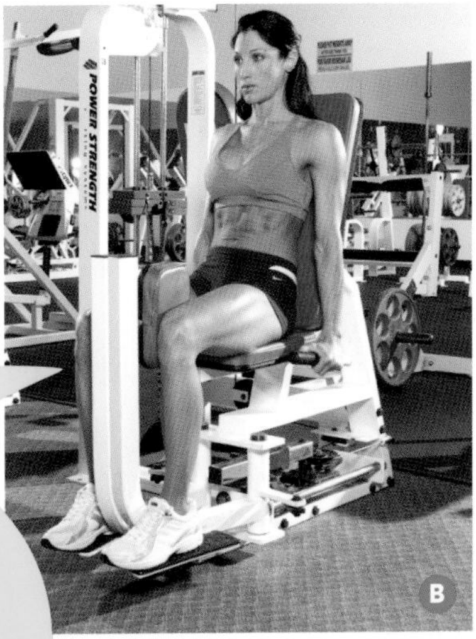


### Inside Edge

***Keep torso upright and stable, using hands to gently assist legs, if necessary, rather than leaning torso to help finish the last couple of reps.***

## Trainer's tips

- Don't overestimate your flexibility when adjusting leg levers for range of motion. Your legs may be able to open beyond hip width in a passive stretch, but generating force in that position puts you at a biomechanical disadvantage, leading to possible groin injury. Back off a few degrees so you can contract inner-thigh muscles more effectively.
- For more inner-thigh isolation, sit with hips slightly forward of the back pad. By completely removing your ability to press back into the pad, you place all of the workload on the inner thighs.
- For an intense superset, follow with plié dumbbell squats.
- To do this move at home, sit on a chair and squeeze a soft stability ball between thighs.

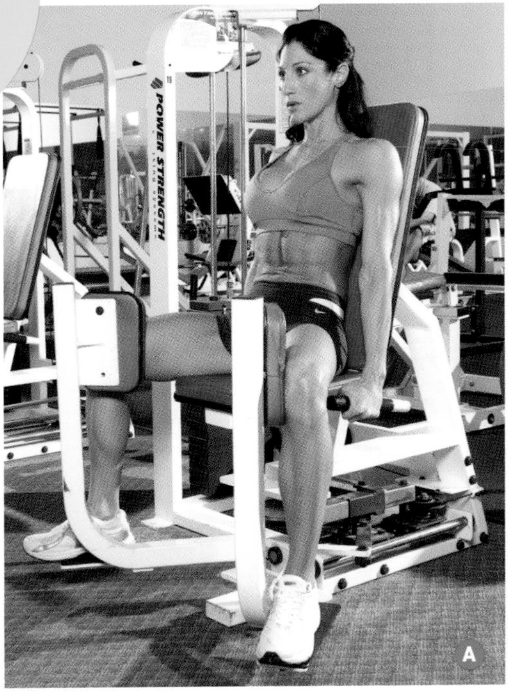

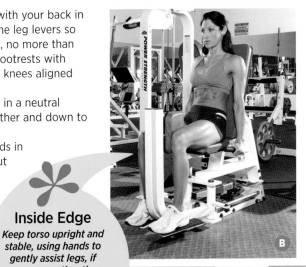

# Seated Leg Curl

BEGINNER/
INTERMEDIATE/ADVANCED

***Muscles Worked:** hamstrings*

## Technique

1. Sit with your entire back against the seat pad. Adjust the seat back to allow the center of your knee to line up with the pivot point of machine, then lower thigh pad to rest on thighs.
2. Adjust the foot bar so it rests just above your heels and against your Achilles tendon; feet are relaxed.
3. Contract abdominal muscles so spine is in a neutral position. Squeeze shoulder blades together and down. Grasp the handrails.
4. Contract your hamstrings to bend knees, bringing heels down and under you in an arc.
5. Hold for two counts, then straighten legs to start position without locking knees.

## Trainer's tips

- Select a weight that allows you to focus on only using the hamstrings to complete the movement; by reducing the weight, the hamstrings may actually be able to work harder.
- Don't contract your calves (which causes them to assist). Using the hip flexors to lift thighs off the pad also reduces the workload.
- Adjust the seat back to line the pivot point of your joint up with the machine's pivot point; this reduces shearing forces at the knee. A properly placed thigh pad will help stabilize the leg for maximum hamstring contraction.
- For variety, switch to a prone lying curl or do the move standing and using a cable.

**Inside Edge**

*Straightening legs slowly to start position keeps tension on the hamstrings, working them eccentrically as well as concentrically.*

A

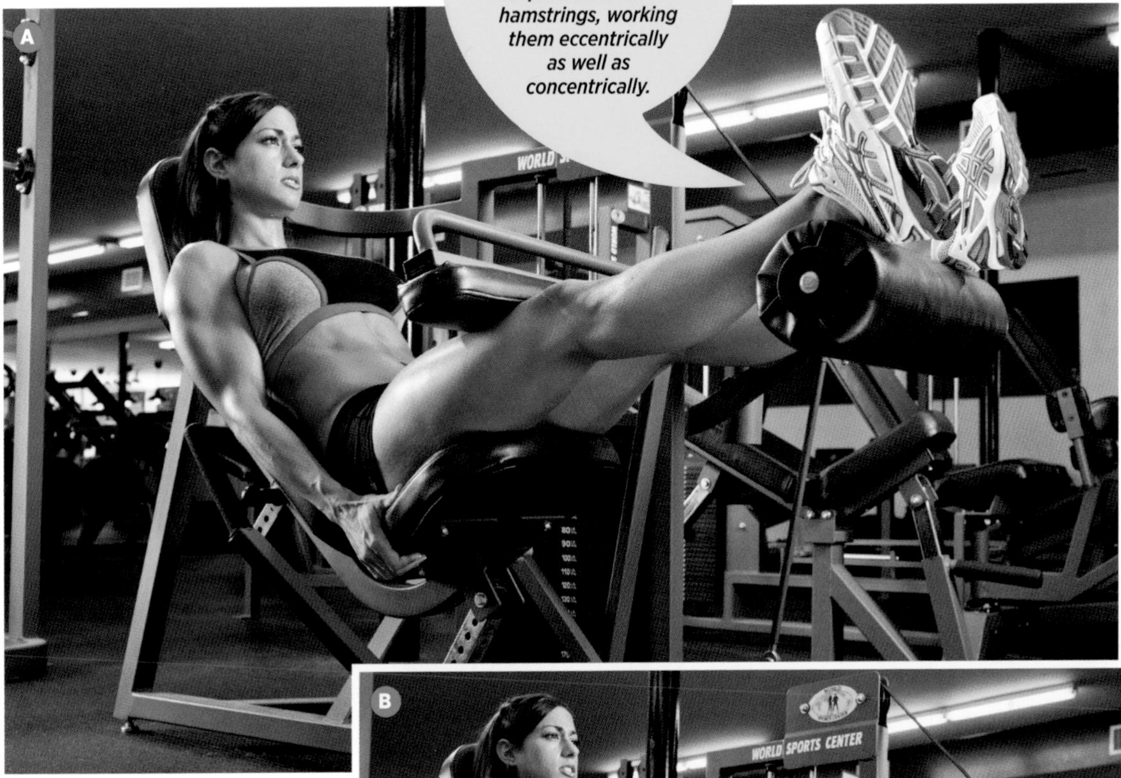

B

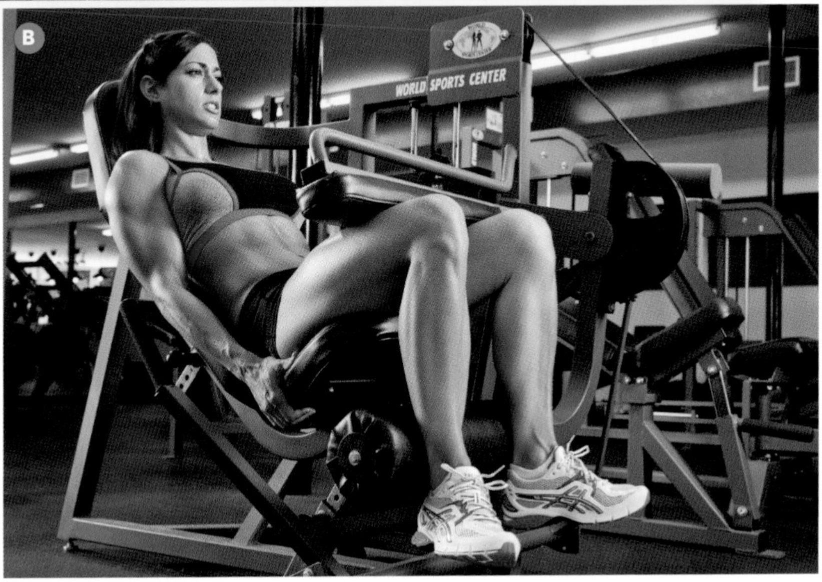

# Side Lunge INTERMEDIATE/ADVANCED

***Muscles Worked:** gluteus maximus, gluteus medius, quadriceps, hamstrings, adductor group, calves; these muscles also work as stabilizers on support leg*

## Technique

1. Hold a light barbell across your upper back, stand with feet slightly apart, legs straight but not locked. (This exercise can also be performed holding dumbbells at the sides.)
2. Contract abdominal muscles so spine is in a neutral position. Squeeze your shoulder blades together and down.
3. Keeping left leg straight, step sideways with right foot, about twice as wide as hips, rotating right leg slightly open from the hip so right toes point out at 45 degrees as you bend right knee, aligning it with second toe.
4. Keep chest lifted and torso centered between both legs; don't lean toward lunging leg.
5. Push back off of right heel, straightening right leg to return to starting position. Repeat for reps or alternate sides.

## Trainer's tips

- Keep torso stable by continuing to retract shoulder blades together throughout the entire movement.
- Don't over-rotate your hip as you step out; your torso and pelvis should remain fairly square.
- Don't allow your lunging leg to go past toes or rotate inward, placing excess stress on knee ligaments and tendons.
- Don't step out so far that you can't push back to start position; this will overstretch the adductors.
- Double the workload by incorporating an upper-body move—such as an overhead shoulder press — with the side lunge.

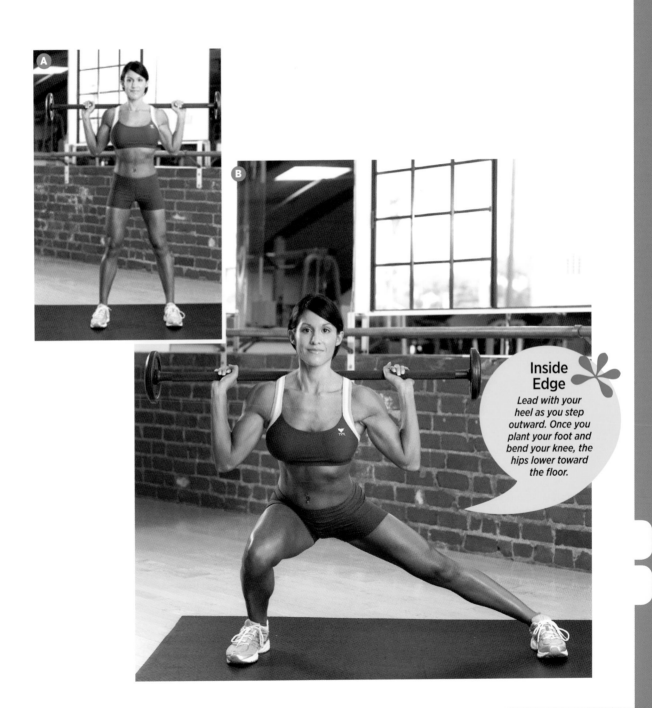


**Inside Edge**

*Lead with your heel as you step outward. Once you plant your foot and bend your knee, the hips lower toward the floor.*

# One-Leg Bench Lunge

INTERMEDIATE/ADVANCED

***Muscles Worked:** gluteus maximus, quadriceps, hamstrings; hip abductors and adductors as stabilizers*

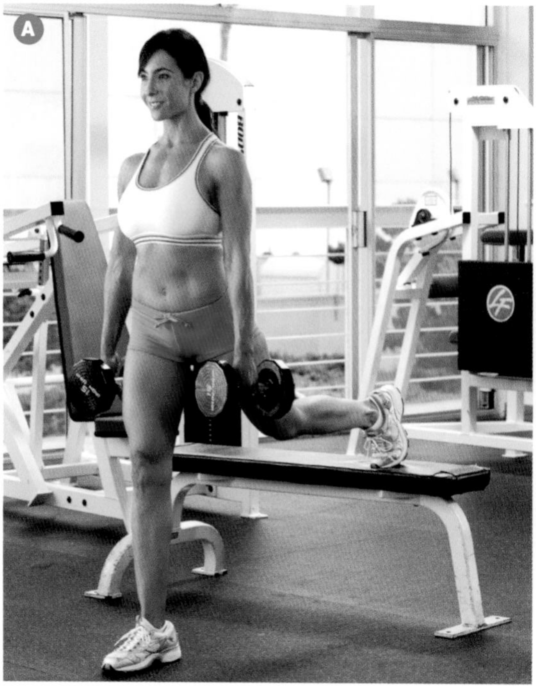


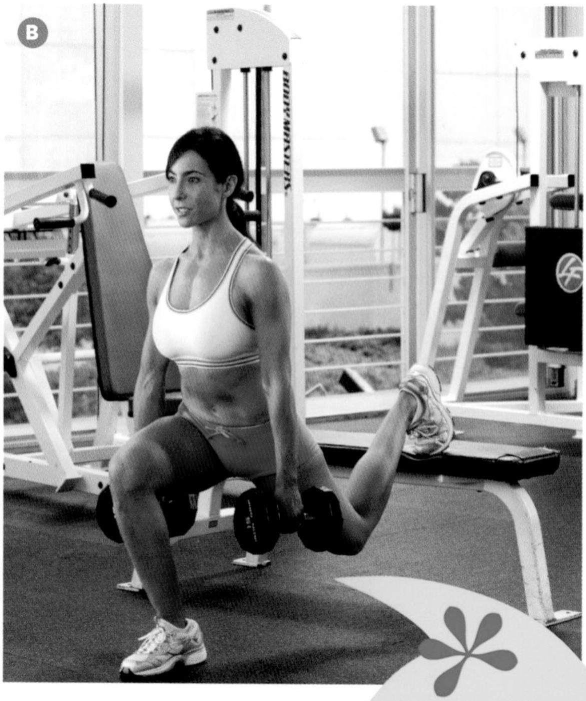


## Technique

1. Holding a dumbbell in each hand, arms hanging by sides and palms facing in, stand with your back to a flat bench, about a stride away. Feet are hip-width apart, legs straight but not locked.
2. Extend one foot behind you, placing toes on bench with knee slightly bent, then adjust position forward to align front knee with ankle.
3. Contract abdominal muscles so spine is in a neutral position. Squeeze shoulder blades together and down.
4. Bend front knee, lowering hips toward floor until angle of front knee approaches 90 degrees and back knee approaches floor.
5. Contract glutes and thighs to straighten legs, returning to start position.
6. Repeat for reps, then switch legs.

## Trainer's tips

- The farther you stand from the bench, and the straighter you keep your back leg, the more challenging the move.
- You may feel more stable with the bench a little closer, especially if you have inflexible hip flexors, which also affect the amount of movement in your hips to bend your back leg.
- Don't press hips forward; continue to drive hips straight up and down.
- Don't let your knee pass your toes.
- For more of a challenge, use a barbell instead of dumbbells or use a stability ball instead of the bench.

### Inside Edge

***Avoid pressing down on the bench with your foot; this will force the glutes and thigh muscles of the front leg to do all the work.***

# Smith Machine Lunge BEGINNER/INTERMEDIATE

***Muscles Worked:** gluteus maximus, quadriceps, hamstrings, calves; hip abductors and adductors as stabilizers*

## Technique

1. Standing in a Smith machine, place bar across upper back and shoulders and hold with an overhand grip wider than shoulders, elbows pointing down.
2. Releasing bar locks, separate legs hip-width apart and take a stride forward with one foot, extending other leg behind you, back heel lifted.
3. Contract abdominal muscles, bringing spine to a neutral position and squeeze shoulder blades together and down.
4. Keeping torso centered between legs and vertical, bend knees, lowering hips toward the floor until knees are bent 90 degrees, front knee aligned over ankle, back knee pointing toward floor.
5. Using glutes, straighten legs to start position.
6. Repeat all reps on one side before switching legs.

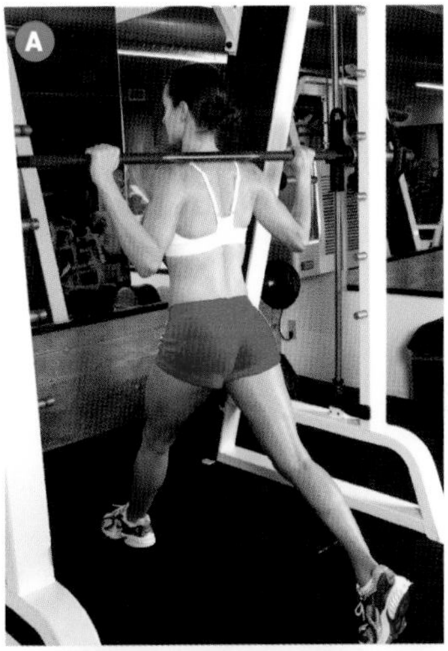


## Trainer's tips

- For optimal safety, make sure you preset the safety catches on each vertical bar.
- To gauge the depth of your lunge, place a bench lengthwise into cage and aim to just clear bench with buttocks at bottom of rep.
- If you experience neck strain, place a bar pad or rolled up towel around bar.
- Try to keep head upright, with neck in line with rest of spine.
- For variety and an intensity boost, alternate legs for each rep; try supersetting with Smith-machine squats; have a partner strip plates for a final drop set; or place one or both feet on an airex pad.

### Inside Edge

***Make sure bar placement allows for proper knee alignment and a vertical spine as you lower. This maximizes effectiveness and reduces the risk of injury.***

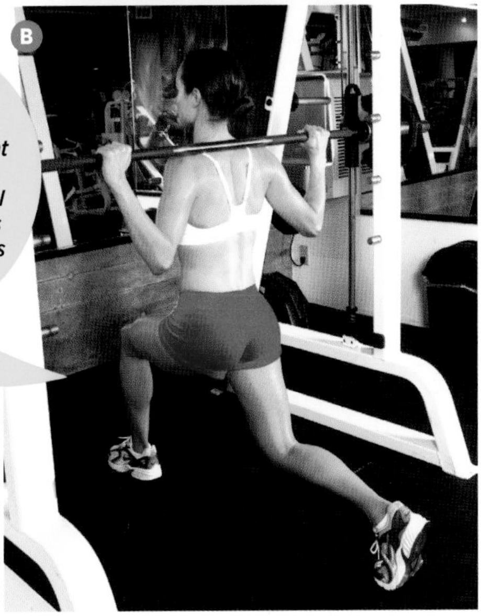

# Squat BEGINNER/INTERMEDIATE/ADVANCED

***Muscles Worked:*** *gluteus maximus, quadriceps, hamstrings; hip abductors and adductors as stabilizers*

## Technique

1. Standing with feet hip-width apart, legs straight but not locked, place a barbell across upper back and shoulders and hold bar with an overhand grip wider than shoulder width, elbows pointing down.
2. Contract abdominal muscles so spine is in a neutral position, and squeeze shoulder blades together and down to stabilize upper back.
3. With bodyweight back toward heels, bend knees and lower hips toward floor, keeping back straight and head aligned with spine until thighs are as parallel to floor as possible, knees approaching 90-degree angles or until you lose your neutral spine position.
4. Using glutes and thigh muscles, drive hips back up, straightening legs to start position in a controlled manner.

## Trainer's tips

- Avoid lower-back problems by paying special attention to your posture as you lower. Check yourself sideways in a mirror without weight to see exactly how far down you can go without rounding your lower back.
- If you have weak hip stabilizers, you may find your knees drifting in toward each other as you descend, especially if you use heavy weight. Keep knees aligned with feet, lowering weight only as far as you can control the descent and ascent.
- For variety, switch to a Smith machine or dumbbells. Superset with exercises like walking lunges and step-up lunges.
- To hit your glutes hard, superset this squat with Romanian deadlifts.

## Inside Edge

*Recruit more glutes, and protect your knees, by keeping bodyweight toward your heels as you lower, pushing through the heels as you stand back up.*

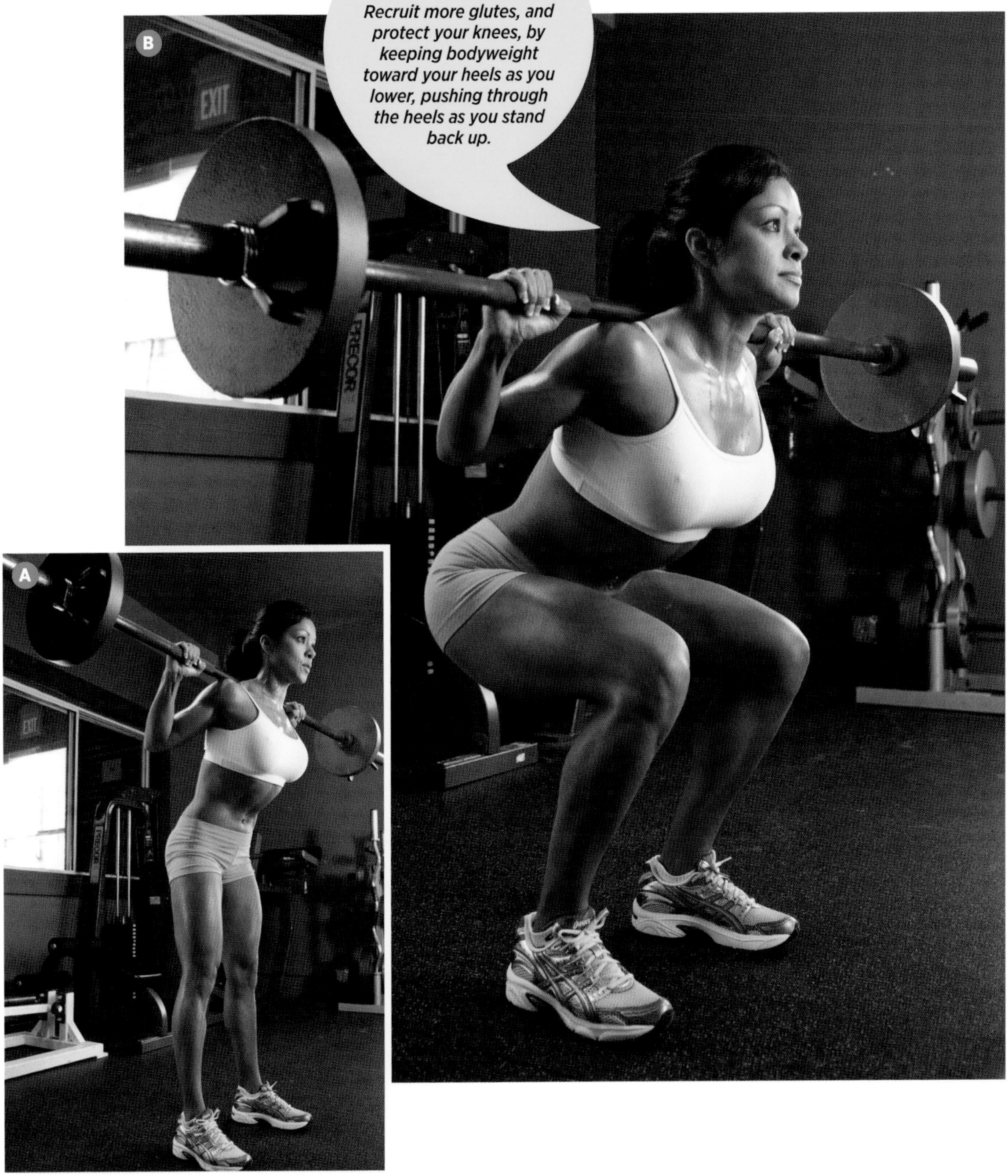

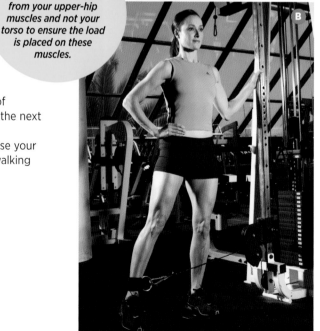

# Standing Cable Abduction

INTERMEDIATE

***Muscles Worked:*** *gluteus maximus, quadriceps, hamstrings, calves; hip abductors and adductors as stabilizers*

## Technique

1. Attach an ankle cuff to a low-cable pulley and place a 10-pound weight about 6 inches away from weight stack.
2. Attach ankle cuff to right ankle, and stand with left foot on plate, knee slightly bent. Lightly grasp bar with left hand for support. Extend right leg across body's midline, keeping shoulders and hips square and level.
3. Contract abdominal muscles so spine is in a neutral position. Squeeze shoulder blades together and down to stabilize upper back.
4. Maintaining position, contract upper hip, lifting right leg out and away from your body, without rotating hips or moving torso.
5. Pause and return to starting position. Repeat for reps, then switch legs.

**Inside Edge**

***Initiate the movement from your upper-hip muscles and not your torso to ensure the load is placed on these muscles.***

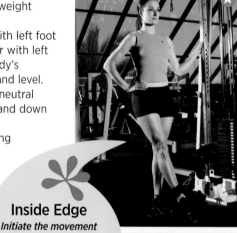

## Trainer's tips

- If you feel lower-back strain, you may be arching your back. Alleviate this by keeping the abs tight and bending the standing knee.
- Experiment with range of motion. In one workout, do only the first half of the range of motion, switching to the second half during the next workout. Finish both with a final drop set.
- Developing the outer hip muscles will increase your stability in more difficult exercises such as walking lunges and dumbbell reverse bench lunges.

# Standing Cable Adduction INTERMEDIATE

***Muscles Worked:*** *hip adductors; gluteus maximus and gluteus medius as stabilizers*

## Technique

1. Attach an ankle cuff to a low-cable pulley and place a 10-pound weight about a foot away from weight stack.
2. Attach ankle cuff to left ankle, and stand with right foot on plate, knee slightly bent. Lightly grasp bar for support with left hand. Extend left leg out toward weight stack, shoulders and hips square, right hand on hip.
3. Contract abdominal muscles so spine is in a neutral position. Squeeze shoulder blades together and down to stabilize upper back.
4. Maintaining position, contract inner-thigh muscles to bring left leg across and slightly in front of right leg without moving torso.
5. Pause and return to starting position. Repeat for reps, then switch legs.

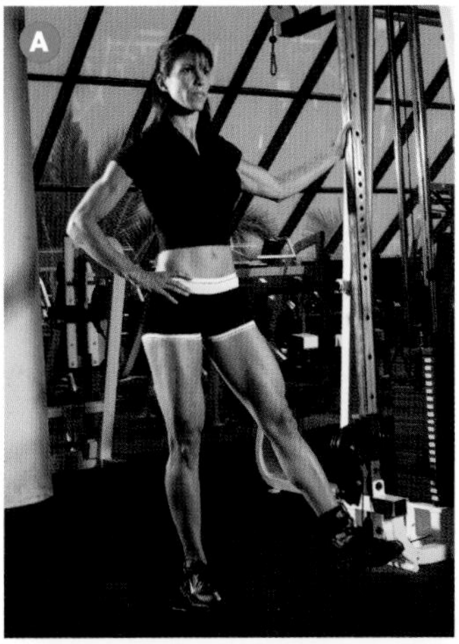


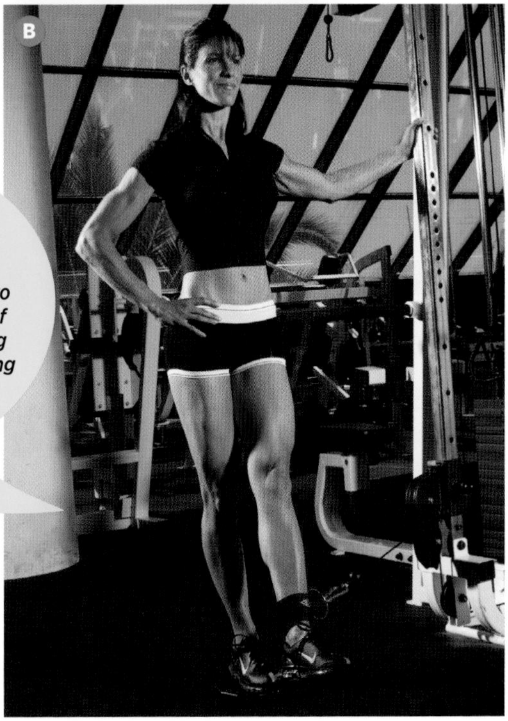


## Trainer's tips

- To increase intensity in the muscle contraction, imagine drawing the insides of the thighs together, pausing at the end of the contraction and squeezing as if trying to hold a pencil between your inner thighs.
- The plate elevates your shoe enough to clear the floor for a smooth movement.
- Keep hips squared and level; don't bring your leg so far across your body that your hips rotate or hike up as you finish.
- At home, use tubing attached to a support, or perform this exercise lying on your side with ankle weight around bottom ankle.

**Inside Edge**

***Don't swing the leg to increase the range of motion. Move the leg smoothly, as if drawing a crescent moon.***

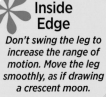

# Stationary Lunge BEGINNER/INTERMEDIATE

***Muscles Worked:*** *gluteus maximus, quadriceps, hamstrings, calves; hip abductors and adductors as stabilizers*

## Technique

1. Standing with feet hip-width apart, hold a dumbbell in each hand, arms hanging by your sides, palms facing in.
2. Take a long stride forward with one foot so you're in a staggered stance, legs straight but not locked and back heel lifted.
3. Center torso between both legs and contract abdominal muscles so spine is in a neutral position. Squeeze shoulder blades together and down to stabilize upper back.
4. Bend knees, lowering hips toward floor until both knees are bent at 90 degrees, front knee aligned over ankle and back knee pointing straight down at floor.
5. Straighten legs to start position. Repeat reps on one side, then switch legs.

## Trainer's tips

- Don't let the front knee drift in as you bend or straighten the leg, which can place stress on ligaments and cartilage. Going a little lighter and slower at first will help keep knee aligned.
- Take a large enough step forward into your staggered stance to keep front knee aligned over ankle.
- By keeping torso upright and breastbone lifted, you can maintain focus on glutes and thighs, and help eliminate any forward torso lean.
- For variety, perform with barbell across upper back and shoulders or stand with front foot in the middle of a length of tubing with handles held at hips.

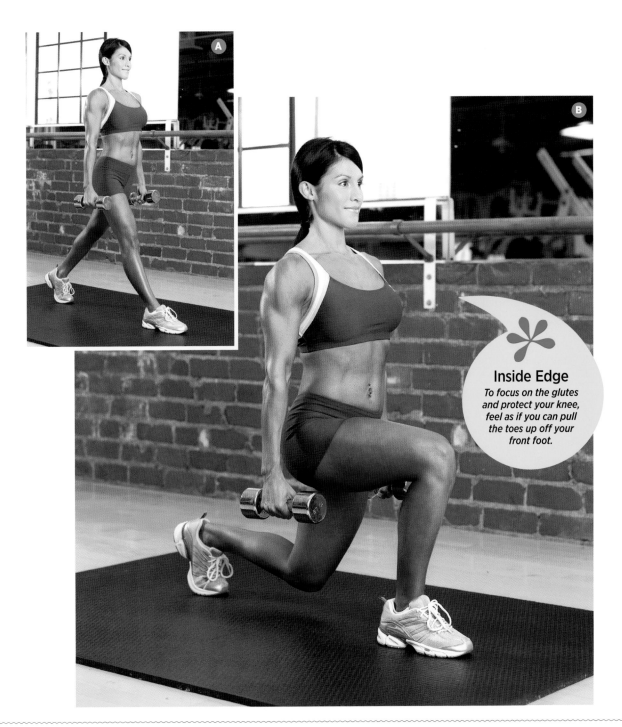

**Inside Edge**

*To focus on the glutes and protect your knee, feel as if you can pull the toes up off your front foot.*

# Step-Up Lunge With Knee Lift ADVANCED

***Muscles Worked:*** *gluteus maximus, quadriceps, hamstrings, calves; gluteus medius and hip adductors as stabilizers*

## Technique

1. Stand facing a weight bench with feet hip-width apart, legs straight but not locked. Hold a dumbbell in each hand, weights in front of shoulders and parallel to floor, palms facing in.
2. Contract abdominal muscles so spine is in a neutral position. Squeeze shoulder blades together and down.
3. Place one foot on top of bench, bending knee and aligning it with ankle. The supporting leg is straight, heel lifted.
4. Bend support knee and push off floor foot to propel body upward, straightening both legs so you're standing on top of bench. Lift knee of support leg to hip height.
5. Step down with lifted foot, softly bending knee to start position.
6. Repeat reps on one side before switching legs.

## Trainer's tips

- Bench height is key: a high bench makes the glutes and thighs work harder, but a bench that's too high can cause torso to lean.
- If the knee lift is too great a challenge, start by just tapping lifted foot on top of bench, then stepping back down, or don't use weight.
- As you push off the floor foot, focus on lifting your entire body upward so when standing on the bench, your shoulders are aligned over hips.

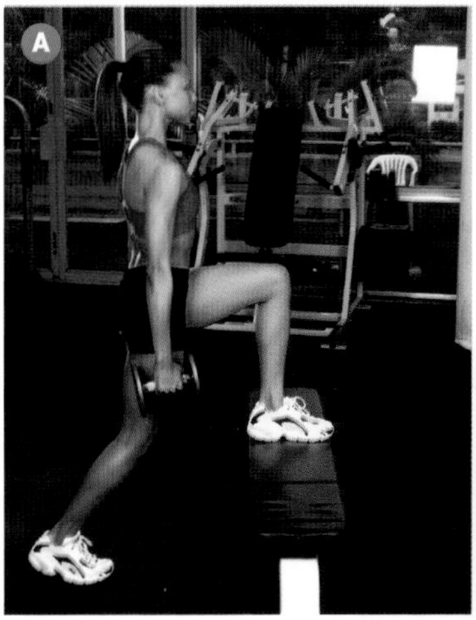


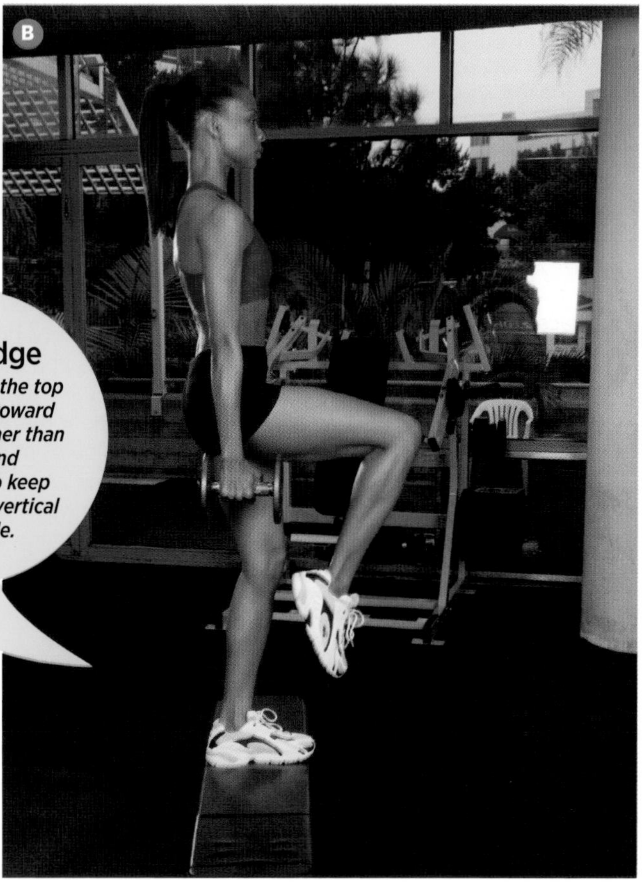


**Inside Edge**

*Imagine lifting the top of your head toward the ceiling, rather than forward and backwards, to keep movement as vertical as possible.*

# Walking Lunge INTERMEDIATE/ADVANCED

***Muscles Worked:*** *gluteus maximus, quadriceps, hamstrings, calves; gluteus medius and hip adductors as stabilizers*

## Technique

1. Holding a dumbbell in each hand, arms hanging down at sides and palms facing in, stand with feet hip-width apart, legs straight but not locked.
2. Contract abdominal muscles so spine is in a neutral position. Squeeze shoulder blades together and down.
3. Keeping torso upright, take a large step forward with one foot, bending both knees and lowering hips toward floor until front knee is bent at 90 degrees. Front thigh is parallel and back knee is pointing down, heel lifted.
4. Straighten both legs, simultaneously pushing off back foot and bringing it up to meet the other. Pause, then repeat with other leg. Continue walking forward to complete set.

## Trainer's tips

- Take a large enough step each time so your front knee stays aligned over ankle and doesn't overshoot toes. Likewise, if your step is too big, you may not be able to step forward without momentum.
- Eliminate any unnecessary arm and torso movement. Don't allow arms to swing forward as you step; keep them at sides at all times. Minimizing torso lean keeps knees aligned with feet.
- For variety, do this exercise with a barbell across upper back and shoulders.
- Use this exercise to spice up your outdoor run/walk program. Run/walk for 5 minutes at moderate pace, 2 minutes at higher intensity, then stop and perform 15–20 walking lunges. Repeat cycle 3–4 times.

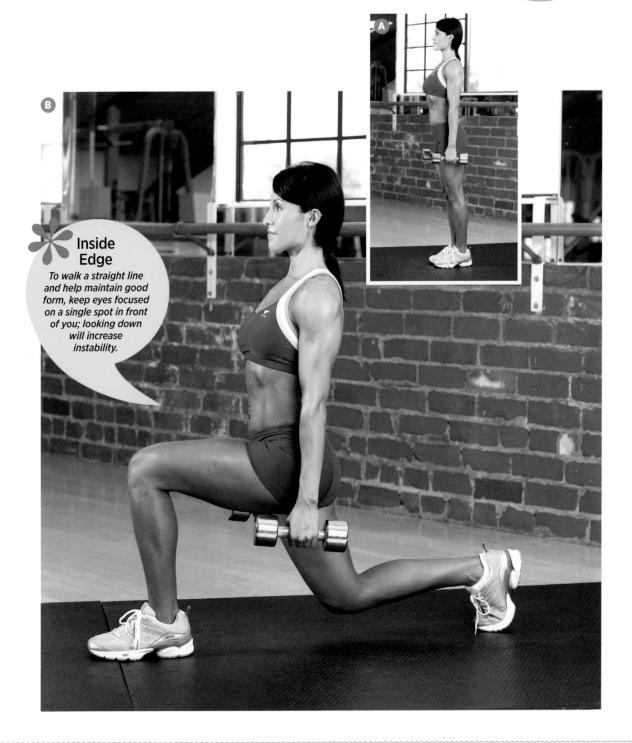


**Inside Edge**

*To walk a straight line and help maintain good form, keep eyes focused on a single spot in front of you; looking down will increase instability.*

## Beginner Workouts

***Directions:*** ***This is a progressive, six-week program using moderate weight. Do the listed exercises twice per week.***

| WEEK | EXERCISE | SETS | REPS |
|---|---|---|---|
| 1 & 2 | Ball Wall Squat | 2 | 12–15 |
| | Stationary Lunge | 2 | 12–15 |
| | Seated Abduction | 2 | 12–15 |
| | Seated Adduction | 2 | 12–15 |
| | Seated Leg Curl | 2 | 12–15 |
| 3 & 4 | Squat | 2 | 12–15 |
| | Smith-Machine Lunge | 1–2 | 10–12 |
| | Plié Dumbbell Squat | 2 | 12–15 |
| | Ball Glute Lift | 1–2 | 10–12 |
| | Seated Abduction | 2 | 12–15 |
| | Seated Adduction | 2 | 12–15 |
| | Seated Leg Curl | 2 | 12–15 |
| 5 & 6 | ***Alternate the following workouts.*** | | |
| | ***Workout 1*** | | |
| | Ball Wall Squat | 1 | 12–15 |
| | Leg Press | 1–2 | 10–12 |
| | Stationary Lunge | 2 | 12–15 |
| | Seated Abduction | 2 | 10–12 |
| | Seated Adduction | 2 | 10–12 |
| | ***Workout 2*** | | |
| | Plié Dumbbell Squat | 1 | 12–15 |
| | Leg Press | 1 | 10–12 |
| | Smith-Machine Lunge | 2 | 12–15 |
| | Seated Leg Curl | 2 | 12–15 |
| | Ball Glute Lift | 1 | 12–15 |

***Notes***

*Rest 45–60 seconds between sets. After six weeks, progress to intermediate workouts if you're ready.*

# Intermediate Workouts

***Directions:*** ***This is a progressive, six-week program using moderate weight. Do the following exercises twice per week.***

| WEEK | EXERCISE | SETS | REPS |
|---|---|---|---|
| 1 & 2 | Leg Press | 3 | 12–15 |
| | Reverse Lunge | 3 | 12–15 |
| | Standing Cable Abduction | 2–3 | 12–15 |
| | Standing Cable Adduction | 2–3 | 12–15 |
| | Plié Dumbbell Squat | 3 | 12–15 |
| | Ball Bridge | 2 | 12–15 |
| | Seated Leg Curl (Drop set)* | 2 | 10/5 |
| 3 & 4 | Plié Dumbbell Squat or Leg Press | 2–3 | 12–15 |
| | Alternating Reverse Bench Lunge | 3 | 10–12 |
| | Romanian Deadlift | 3 | 10–12 |
| | Side Lunge (same side) | 2–3 | 12–15 |
| | ***Superset:*** | 2 | |
| | Squat | | 8–10 |
| | Jump Squat | | 8–10 |
| | Ball Glute Lift | 1–2 | 10–15 |
| 5 & 6 | ***Alternate the following workouts.*** | | |
| | ***Workout 1*** | | |
| | Cable Kickback | 1 | 15–20 |
| | ***Superset:*** | 2 | |
| | Leg Press | | 12–15 |
| | Walking Lunge | | 12–15 |
| | ***Superset:*** | 2–3 | |
| | Romanian Deadlift | | 10–12 |
| | Ball Bridge Curl | | 10–12 |
| | Cable Kickback | 1 | 15–20 |
| | ***Workout 2*** | | |
| | Smith-Machine Lunge (Alternate Legs) | 2–3 | 10–12 |
| | One-Leg Bench Squat | 2 | 12–15 |
| | ***Superset (same leg):*** | 2 | 12–15 |
| | Standing Cable Abduction<br>Standing Cable Adduction | | |
| | Plié Dumbbell Squat | 2–3 | 10–12 |
| | Seated Leg Curl** | 1st | 12–15 |
| | ***For pyramid sets, increase weight* | *2nd* | *10–12* |
| | *as you decrease reps.* | *3rd* | *8–10* |

**Notes**

*Rest 60–90 seconds between sets. After 6 weeks, progress to advanced workouts if you're ready.*
**For drop sets, reduce weight enough to complete 5 more reps.*

# Advanced Workouts

***Directions:* Perform two workouts a week, choosing from the following programs.**

| EXERCISE | SETS | REPS |
|---|---|---|
| ***Workout 1*** | | |
| ***Superset:*** | 3 | |
| Squat | | 8–10 |
| Walking Lunge | | 10–12 |
| Step-Up Lunge With Knee Lift | | 10–12 |
| ***Superset:*** | 3 | |
| Jump Squat | | 12–15 |
| Romanian Deadlift | | 10–12 |
| Leg Press | 1st | 8–10 |
| (decrease weight as you increase | 2nd | 8–10 |
| reps) | 3rd | 12–15 |
| | 4th | 12–15 |
| ***Workout 2*** | | |
| ***Superset:*** | 3 | |
| Plié Dumbbell Squat | | 12–15 |
| Standing Cable Abduction | | 12–15 |
| Standing Cable Adduction | | 12–15 |
| ***Superset:*** | 3 | |
| Reverse Lunge (same side) | | 10–12 |
| Step-Up Lunge With Knee Lift (same side) | | 10–12 |
| Seated Leg Curl | 1st | 12–15 |
| (Drop set 2nd and 3rd sets)* | 2nd | 10/5 |
| | 3rd | 10/5 |
| ***Workout 3*** | | |
| Leg Press | 3 | 30 (10 with parallel legs, 10 with plié stance, 10 with feet together) |
| ***Superset:*** | 3 | |
| Alternating Reverse Bench Lunge | | 12–15 |
| Cable Kickback | | 12–15 |
| ***Superset:*** | 3 | |
| Side Lunge (alternate sides) | | 12–15 |
| Romanian Deadlift | | 8–10 |
| ***Superset:*** | 3 | |
| Ball Bridge | | 10–12 |
| Ball Bridge Curl | | 10–12 |

**Notes**

*Rest 60–90 seconds between sets or supersets. *For drop sets, reduce weight enough to perform five additional reps.*

# Can't-Get-to-the-Gym Workouts

***Directions:** Do one of the following workouts when you want to work out at home or on the road. Change the order for variety.*

| EXERCISE | SETS | REPS |
|---|---|---|
| *Workout 1* | | |
| Plié Dumbbell Squat* | 2-3 | 12-15 |
| Romanian Deadlift | 2-3 | 12-15 |
| Stationary Lunge* or Walking Lunge | 2-3 | 12-15 |
| Squat* or Jump Squat | 2-3 | 10-15 |
| *Workout 2* | | |
| Ball Wall Squat* or Squat | 2-3 | 12-15 |
| Reverse Lunge* or | 2-3 | 10-15 |
| ***Superset:*** | 2-3 | |
| Reverse Lunge | | 12-15 |
| Step-up Lunge With Knee Lift | | 12-15 |
| Side Lunge | 2-3 | 10-12 |
| Ball Glute Lift* | 2-3 | 12-15 |
| ***Superset:*** | 2-3 | |
| Ball Bridge | | 10-15 |
| Ball Bridge Curl | | 10-15 |

**Notes**

*Rest 60–90 seconds between sets. If you're a beginner, only do the exercises marked with an asterisk (*).*

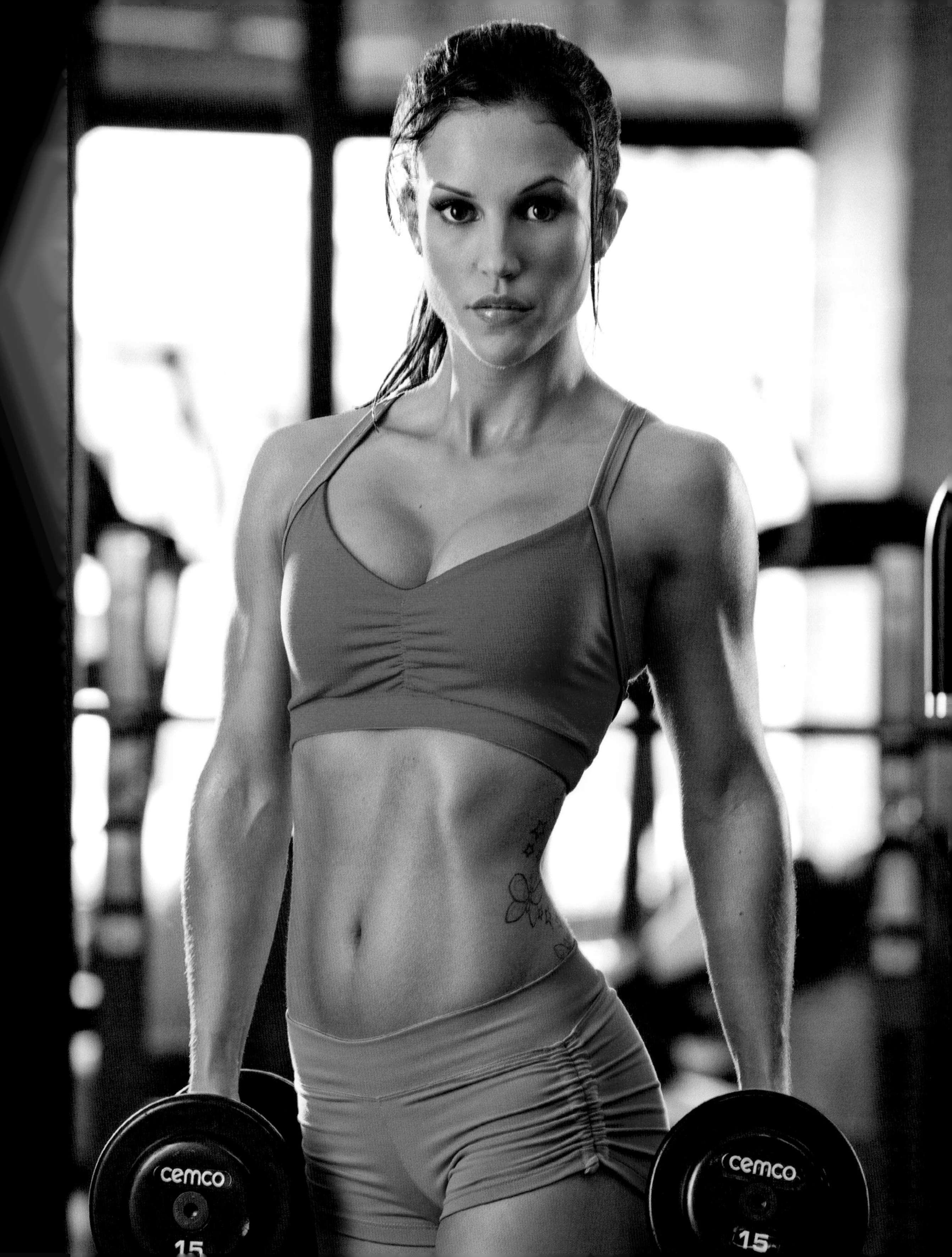
cemco
15
cemco
15

Chapter 8

# Shoulders

*Cap off your toned physique with flawless delts.*

THE DELTOIDS ARE THE TRIANGULAR MUSCLES that give shape and roundness to your shoulders. The deltoids comprise three heads that have different origins but insert at the same place on your upper arm. The anterior head at the front of your shoulder attaches on your collarbone and helps raise your arm up and forward and rotate it inward. The posterior head is at the rear and attaches on your shoulder blade to move your arm toward the rear and rotate it outward. The lateral head, which is between the other two, lifts your arm to the side and helps the anterior and posterior heads in their movements. The trapezius, an upper back muscle that moves your shoulder blades, is an accessory muscle to the deltoids that works in any overhead pressing motion.

## General Guidelines for TRAINING SHOULDERS

***Be sure to include compound exercises that train multiple heads at once.***

Avoid using your bodyweight to hoist the weight or to lift it higher; using momentum doesn't contribute to the effectiveness of any exercise.

Shoulders are especially vulnerable to injury, so always start with a warm-up set to ensure the joints are supple and ready for a training session.

For a well-rounded shoulder program, be sure to include compound exercises that train multiple heads at once as well as isolation exercises that target different portions of your deltoids.

You may find that you can get more out of your shoulder work by regularly varying reps and weight. More often, working with light to moderate rather than heavy weight and doing more reps is safer, particularly when doing overhead pressing movements. This type of regimen gives the shoulder muscles a finer, more defined cut than working with heavy weights.

Try using dumbbells instead of a barbell or cables. Using different equipment trains your three-headed deltoids at different angles, making your workouts more effective.

# Barbell Overhead Press ADVANCED

***Muscles Worked:*** *lateral and anterior deltoid; upper fibers of trapezius; upper fibers of pectoralis major; lower fibers of trapezius and rhomboids as stabilizers*

## Technique

1. Standing with feet hip-width apart, legs straight but not locked, hold a barbell at shoulder height, elbows bent and pointing toward floor, forearms parallel to each other, wrists straight and palms facing forward.
2. Balance your bodyweight so it's evenly distributed between toes and heels of both feet.
3. Contract abdominal muscles to bring spine to a neutral position; chest is lifted, shoulders are relaxed.
4. Press shoulder blades together and down, then straighten arms overhead without locking elbows or cocking wrists; keep barbell in your peripheral vision at the top of the lift.
5. Slowly bend elbows, and lower barbell to start position.

## Trainer's tips

- Keep torso upright and vertical; don't let the weight of the barbell force you to lean backwards, placing stress on your spine.
- Don't use a weight so heavy that you have to cock your wrist backwards in order to hold it.
- Always keep the bar in front of you, never behind the neck.
- Don't rest the bar directly on your collarbone.
- If you've never lifted a barbell overhead, start by sitting with your back supported against an incline bench adjusted to 90 degrees.

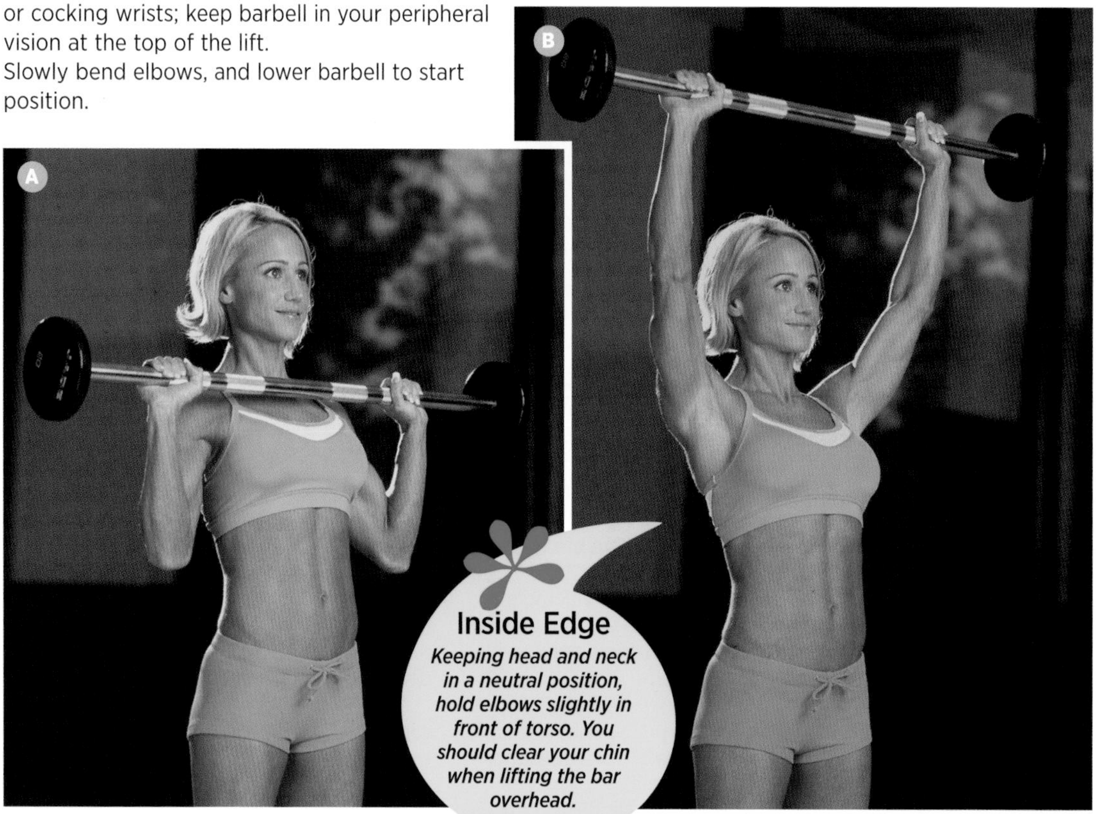


**Inside Edge**

*Keeping head and neck in a neutral position, hold elbows slightly in front of torso. You should clear your chin when lifting the bar overhead.*

# Bent-Over High Row ADVANCED

***Muscles Worked:*** *posterior deltoid; middle and lower trapezius; rhomboids; upper fibers of latissimus dorsi; erector spinae and abdominals as stabilizers*

## Technique

1. Holding a barbell with straight arms in an overhand grip, hands slightly wider than shoulder-width apart, stand with feet separated hip-width apart, legs straight but not locked, bar in front of you close to thighs.
2. Squeeze shoulder blades together and down to stabilize spine, contract abdominal muscles and bend knees, flexing forward at hips. Keep back straight until it's almost parallel to the floor and arms hang, with barbell at shin level and in line with shoulders.
3. Maintain bent-over position, keeping back muscles lengthened, head and neck in line with spine.
4. Keeping wrists straight, bend elbows and pull bar up until it touches lower rib cage, then slowly straighten arms to start position.

**Inside Edge**

***Contract your rear delts as you lift the bar; this helps the delts work in tandem with your upper back muscles to initiate the lift.***

## Trainer's tips

- Keep back in the same position as you lift the bar. Raising your torso as you lift the bar can place stress on your entire back.
- Look down but don't drop your head, which can strain your neck and pull on upper back muscles, affecting your ability to keep shoulder blades pulled back and down.
- In the bent-over position, don't let your abs sag, which can cause you to lose torso stability as well as put pressure on your spine.
- For variety, do this exercise with dumbbells or perform a standing bent-over flye to get deeper into the rear delts.

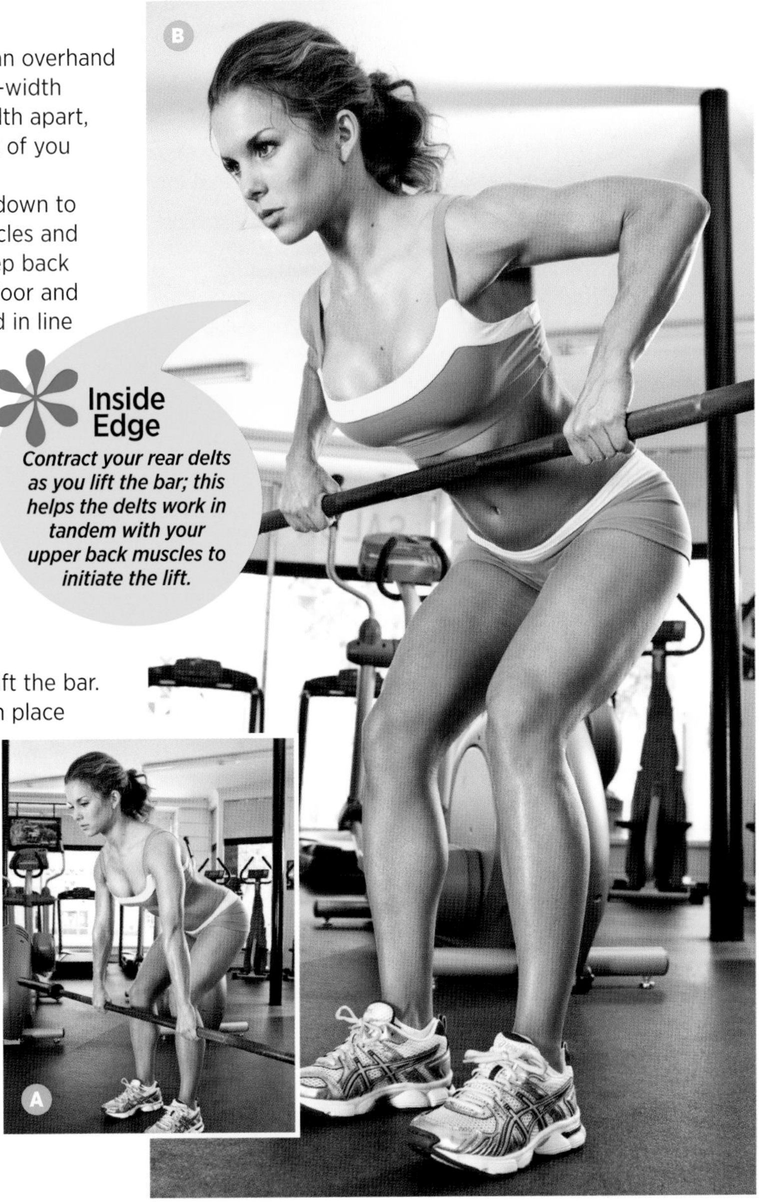

# Bent-Over Standing Rear Flye

INTERMEDIATE/ADVANCED

***Muscles Worked:*** *posterior deltoid; rhomboids; middle trapezius; erector spinae and abdominals as stabilizers*

## Technique

1. Standing with feet hip-width apart, hold a dumbbell in each hand, arms by your sides. Bend your knees, then flex forward from your hips until your back is parallel to the floor. Let arms hang straight down in line with shoulders, elbows in a slight arc, palms facing in, wrists neutral.
2. Draw shoulder blades down and together, moving ears away from shoulders, head and neck aligned with spine.
3. Maintain this position and contract upper back muscles to lift arms up and out to the sides until elbows are even with shoulders. Keep wrists neutral through the entire movement.
4. Pause, then slowly lower dumbbells to start position and repeat.

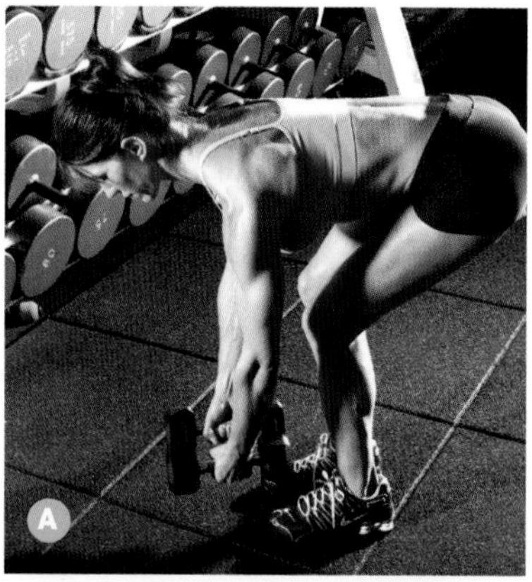
A

## Trainer's tips

- Keep back parallel and straight. Rounding your back as you lift puts stress on your spine, particularly the discs and connective tissue.
- To get into the correct bent-over position, bend knees enough so you feel your back lengthen, then slightly lift your tailbone by extending your hamstrings.
- Lift arms out and up in an arc but don't throw arms up to get more height; this overstretches pectoral tissue and stresses the shoulder joint and its attachments.

### Inside Edge

***Use your back muscles to initiate the movement rather than just lifting your arms. Your arms will naturally lift to the proper height with less effort.***

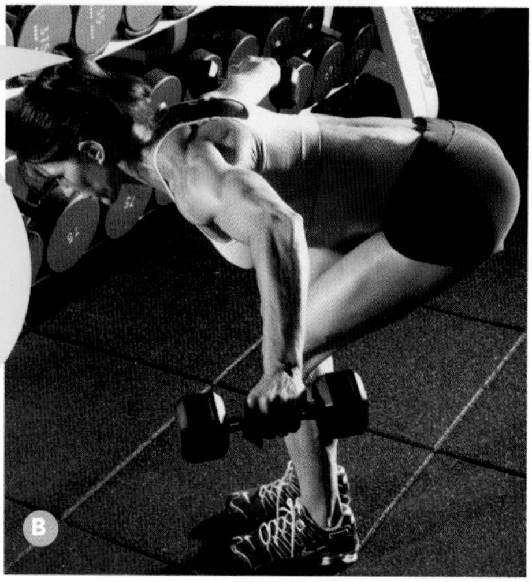
B

# Front Raise

**BEGINNER/INTERMEDIATE/ADVANCED**

***Muscles Worked:*** *anterior deltoid; lower trapezius and rhomboids as stabilizers*

## Technique

1. Holding a dumbbell in each hand with arms hanging in front of your thighs and palms facing back, stand with your feet about hip-width apart, legs straight but not locked and bodyweight balanced between toes and heels.
2. Contract abdominal muscles so spine is in a neutral position, squeeze shoulder blades together and down to stabilize upper back. Keep chest lifted, shoulders down and chin level.
3. Raise both arms up and in front of you to shoulder height, no higher, keeping wrists straight and forearms parallel.
4. Pause, then slowly lower to start position while maintaining a strong torso and without rolling shoulders forward.

**Inside Edge**

***Think of lifting the dumbbells forward and then up as opposed to just straight up; this will innervate more delt fibers and enhance results.***

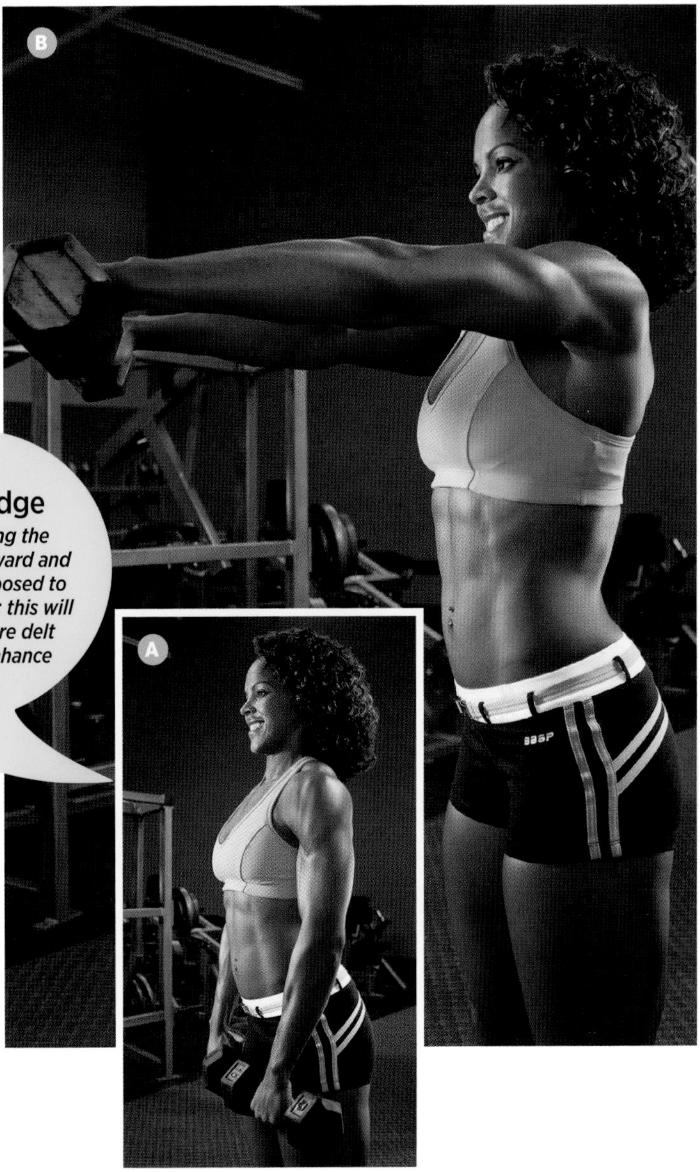


## Trainer's tips

- Don't lean backwards as you lift the weights; it's easy to fall back on your heels, especially if you're trying to lift more weight.
- Use a weight that will challenge you, but not one so heavy that you can't lift to shoulder height for each rep.
- Your arm should be one lever from shoulder joint to knuckles, and wrists should be straight (neutral). Dropping your wrists strains the forearm muscles.
- Initiate the lift from your front shoulders, and continue to draw shoulder blades down as you lift.
- For variety, alternate and lift one arm at a time.
- For more of a challenge, try using a barbell.

# Incline Side-Lying Raise INTERMEDIATE

***Muscles Worked:** lateral deltoid*

## Technique

1. Adjust an incline bench to a 30–45-degree angle and kneel sideways on bench, bending both knees and keeping them together to stack your hips and shoulders. Keep neck in line with the rest of the body.
2. Hold a dumbbell with top arm and rest hip in line with shoulder, elbow in a soft arc, palm down.
3. Contract abdominal muscles so spine is in a neutral position and your body forms one line on the bench from shoulders to hips.
4. Squeeze shoulder blades together and down, then lift arm up past parallel to the floor.
5. Pause then lower to start position. Repeat for reps then switch sides.

## Trainer's tips

- At the beginning of every rep, pull the entire shoulder blade area down and together before moving your arm. Keep shoulders down and don't let them move up around ears when you lift.
- Use a weight you can lift and move through a full range of motion but no higher than shoulders; if you lift any higher than shoulder height, there is no more applied resistance on the muscle.
- Keep elbow in a soft arc, initiating the lift from your middle shoulder, without rotating shoulder, and turning dumbbell up to get more height.
- For variety, do either a seated or standing lateral raise.

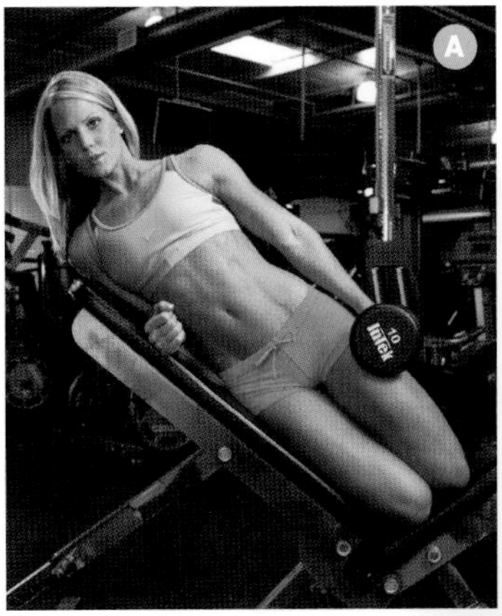

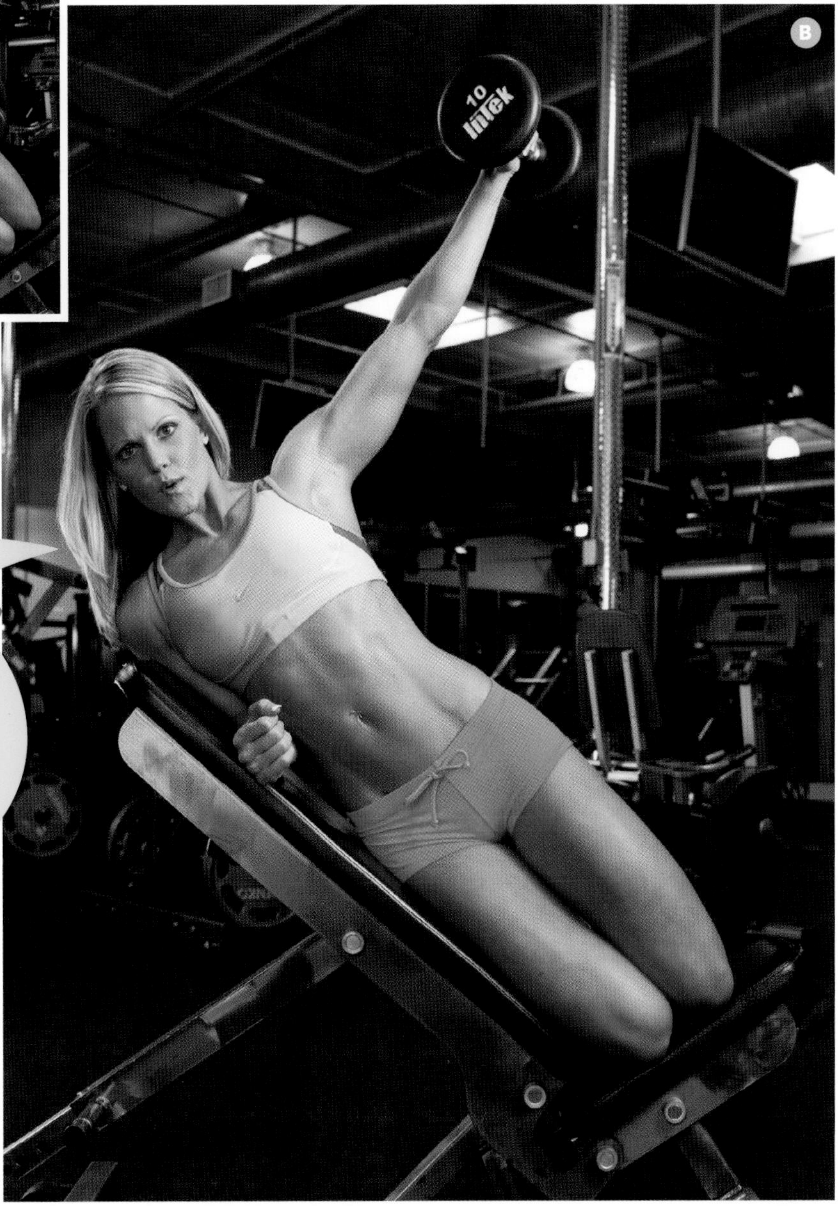

### Inside Edge

*Keep your elbow in a fixed position so all the movement is executed by the lateral deltoid during both the lifting and lowering phases.*

# Prone Flye BEGINNER/INTERMEDIATE

***Muscles Worked:*** *posterior deltoid; rhomboids; middle trapezius; erector spinae and abdominals as stabilizers*

## Technique

1. Lie facedown on a incline bench, with chin just over the bench edge, legs extended toward the floor.
2. Hold a dumbbell in each hand, arms hanging straight down and aligned with shoulders, keeping a bend in the elbows so dumbbells are raised, palms facing in toward the bench.
3. Contract abdominal muscles, dropping tailbone down so spine is in a neutral position, hipbones against the bench.
4. Squeeze shoulder blades together and down, and slightly elevate chest. Lift arms up and out to your sides to shoulder height, palms facing down at top of the movement.
5. Pause, then slowly lower arms to start position.

## Trainer's tips

- Use your back muscles to initiate the movement, then let arms follow.
- To better target the rear delts, gently press shoulders and elbows out at the top of the movement. Although it's a very small movement, it does a lot for shoulder development.
- Keep your tailbone pulled downward so hips stay on the bench and you don't "inchworm" and arch your back; keeping your abs tight will help you successfully maintain this position.
- Don't lift arms any higher than shoulder height in this prone position — doing so could strain shoulder and pec tissue.
- For variety, do this exercise using an decline bench; or, if you're more advanced, try it bent over and standing.

**Inside Edge**

*Continue squeezing shoulder blades together for the entire movement. At the top, pause for a final peak contraction of both mid back and rear deltoid muscles.*

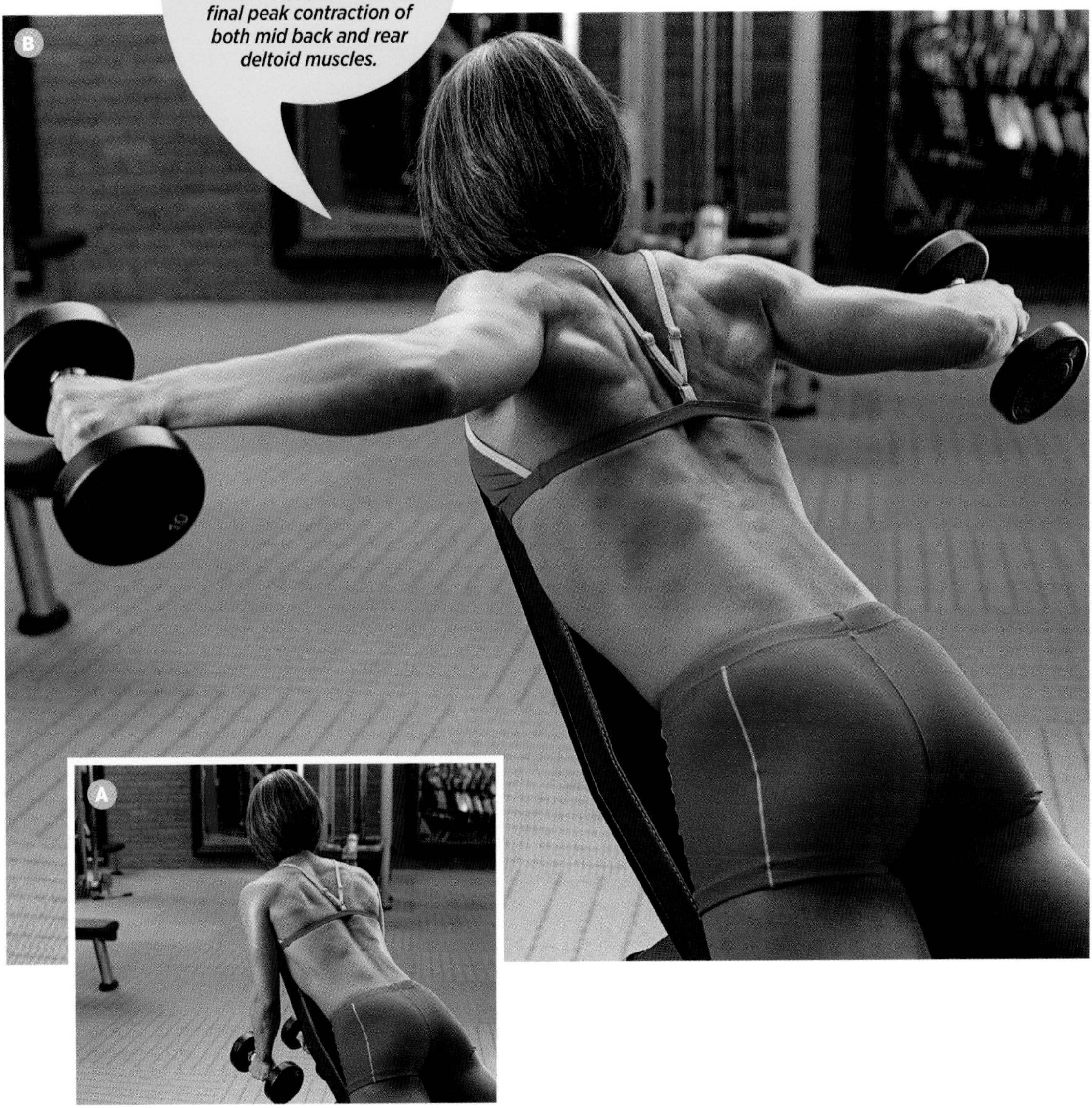

# Seated Dumbbell Lateral Raise

BEGINNER/INTERMEDIATE

***Muscles Worked:** lateral deltoid; trapezius and rhomboids as stabilizers*

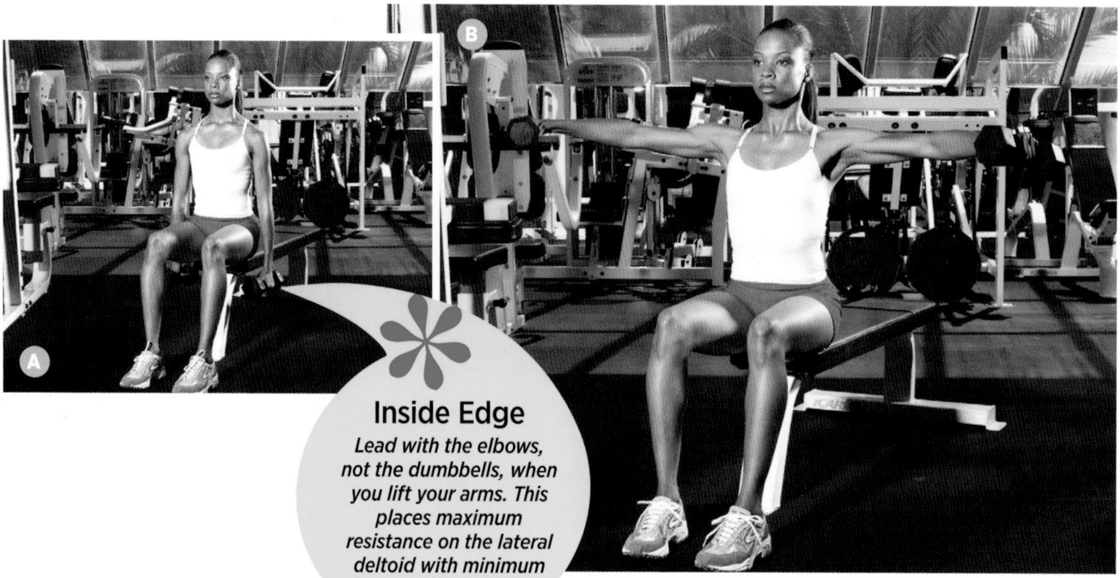


**Inside Edge**

***Lead with the elbows, not the dumbbells, when you lift your arms. This places maximum resistance on the lateral deltoid with minimum stress.***

## Technique

1. Holding a dumbbell in each hand, arms hanging at your sides with a slight arc to elbows and palms facing in, sit on the end of a flat bench, knees bent and aligned with ankles, feet flat on floor.
2. Contract abdominal muscles, bringing spine to a neutral position. Draw shoulder blades together and down to stabilize position. Keep chest lifted, neck and shoulders relaxed.
3. Maintain erect posture and lift arms up and out until they're parallel to the floor, palms facing down, wrists neutral.
4. Pause at the top of the lift, then slowly lower arms to start position.

## Trainer's tips

- Keep an arclike pattern to the arm lift to ensure the middle deltoid does all the work; with arms straight, it's easy to lock elbows or lift from your wrists.
- Keep your shoulders down and away from your ears so your arms can move through a full range of motion.
- Don't use momentum to get arms above shoulder height; this stresses the shoulder joint and rotator cuff muscles.
- Don't roll arms over: If you look over your shoulder, your lateral deltoid should be visible and centered.
- For more support, sit with your back against an incline bench adjusted to 90 degrees.
- For more of a challenge, do this exercise standing.

# Seated Machine Press BEGINNER

***Muscles Worked:*** *lateral and anterior deltoid; upper fibers of trapezius; upper fibers of pectoralis major; lower fibers of trapezius and rhomboids as stabilizers*

## Technique

1. Adjust a shoulder-press machine so handles are at or just above shoulder level. Sit into the seat so that your lower back is fully supported by the back pad, knees bent and in line with ankles, feet flat on floor. (Depending on machine, you can cross ankles or place feet on a bench.)
2. Contract abdominal muscles so spine is in a neutral position, then grasp the handles with an overhand grip, making sure shoulders, elbows and wrists are all in line.
3. Press handles up, fully extending arms overhead without locking elbows.
4. Pause at the top before slowly returning to the start position.

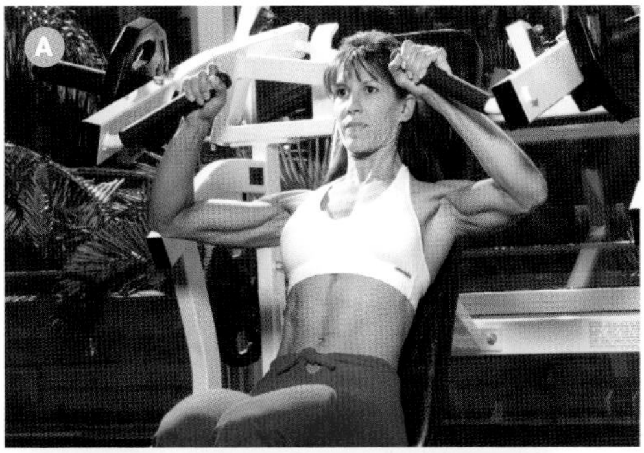


## Trainer's tips

- Maintain a neutral spine: Don't press back into pad or arch your back in order to lift more weight.
- Keep shoulders back and down, and chest lifted to facilitate shoulder and back work.
- Make sure the seat isn't too far forward to start, impinging the shoulder; your elbows should point down and the bars should align with the center of your shoulders.
- Vary your grip to work the muscles a little differently.
- For more of a challenge, do this exercise seated or standing using free dumbbells or a barbell.

**Inside Edge**

***The machine will stabilize your torso so you can safely lift weights that are a little heavier.***

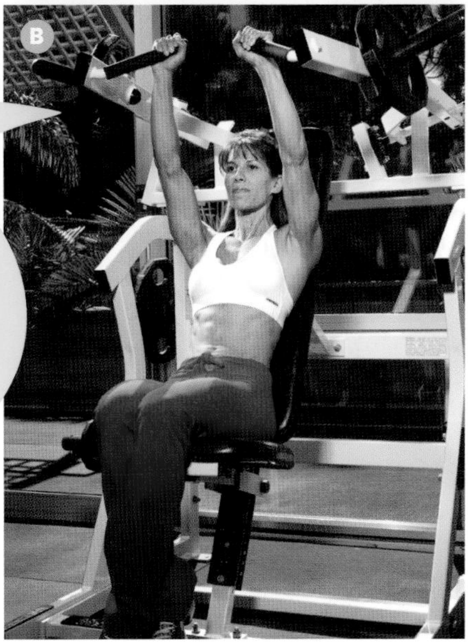

# Seated Dumbbell Overhead Press BEGINNER

***Muscles Worked:** lateral and anterior deltoid; upper fibers of trapezius; upper fibers of pectoralis major; lower fibers of trapezius and rhomboids as stabilizers*

## Technique

1. Sit on a low-back seat (for more support use an incline bench with back adjusted to 90 degrees and press back against back pad) and hold a dumbbell in each hand at shoulder height. Elbows are bent, forearms parallel, wrists straight and palms face each other.
2. Separate feet hip-width apart and bend knees, placing feet flat on floor and aligning knees over ankles.
3. Contract abdominal muscles to bring spine to a neutral position; chest is lifted, shoulders relaxed.
4. Press shoulder blades together and down, then straighten arms overhead, rotating palms forward at the top of the lift, without locking elbows or cocking wrists. Keep weights in your peripheral vision.
5. Slowly bend elbows, lowering to start position.

## Trainer's tips

- As you press arms overhead, protect your shoulder joint by keeping weights in line with shoulders rather than pressing them together at the top.
- Fully extend arms without locking elbows. Don't lean backwards or tuck your tailbone.
- Use moderate weight when pressing overhead to protect the delicate shoulder joint.

**Inside Edge**

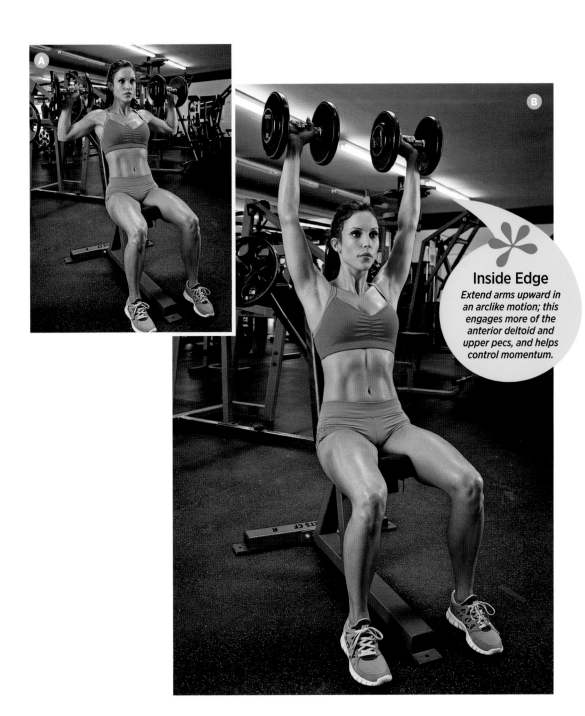

*Extend arms upward in an arclike motion; this engages more of the anterior deltoid and upper pecs, and helps control momentum.*

# Standing Dumbbell Lateral Raise

INTERMEDIATE/ADVANCED

***Muscles Worked:** lateral deltoid; middle and lower fibers of trapezius and rhomboids as stabilizers*

## Technique

1. Holding a dumbbell in each hand, arms hanging by your sides and palms facing in, stand with feet hip-width apart, knees slightly bent, weight balanced evenly between toes and heels. Maintain a slight arc to your elbows, wrists in a neutral position.
2. Contract your abdominal muscles so spine is in a neutral position; keep chest lifted, shoulders down and relaxed, neck long and chin level.
3. Keeping the slight arc in your elbows, lift arms up and out to your sides until they're at shoulder height, no higher, keeping dumbbells level, palms down and wrists straight at the top of the movement.
4. Pause, then slowly lower arms to start position.

## Trainer's tips

- Use a weight that allows you to isolate your shoulders to initiate the movement. You should be able to pause at the top without immediately dropping your arms.
- Keep your torso lifted and don't scrunch your shoulders up around your ears or round your back. If any of these mistakes occur, you may need to lighten your weight or try the seated version.
- For variety, try tilting the dumbbells slightly forward and down as if you're pouring water from pitchers at the top of the movement. Or, to protect your shoulders, lead the movement with thumbs up.

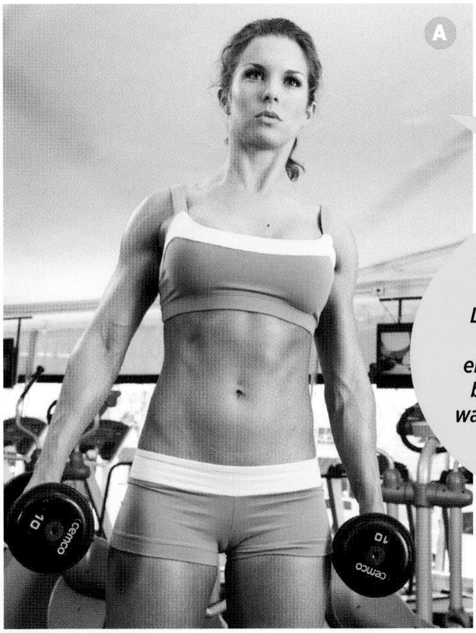


## Inside Edge

*Lead the movement upward from your elbows as if you were balancing a glass of water on each shoulder and trying not to spill.*

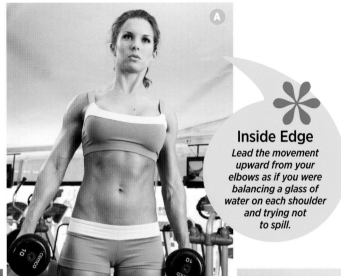

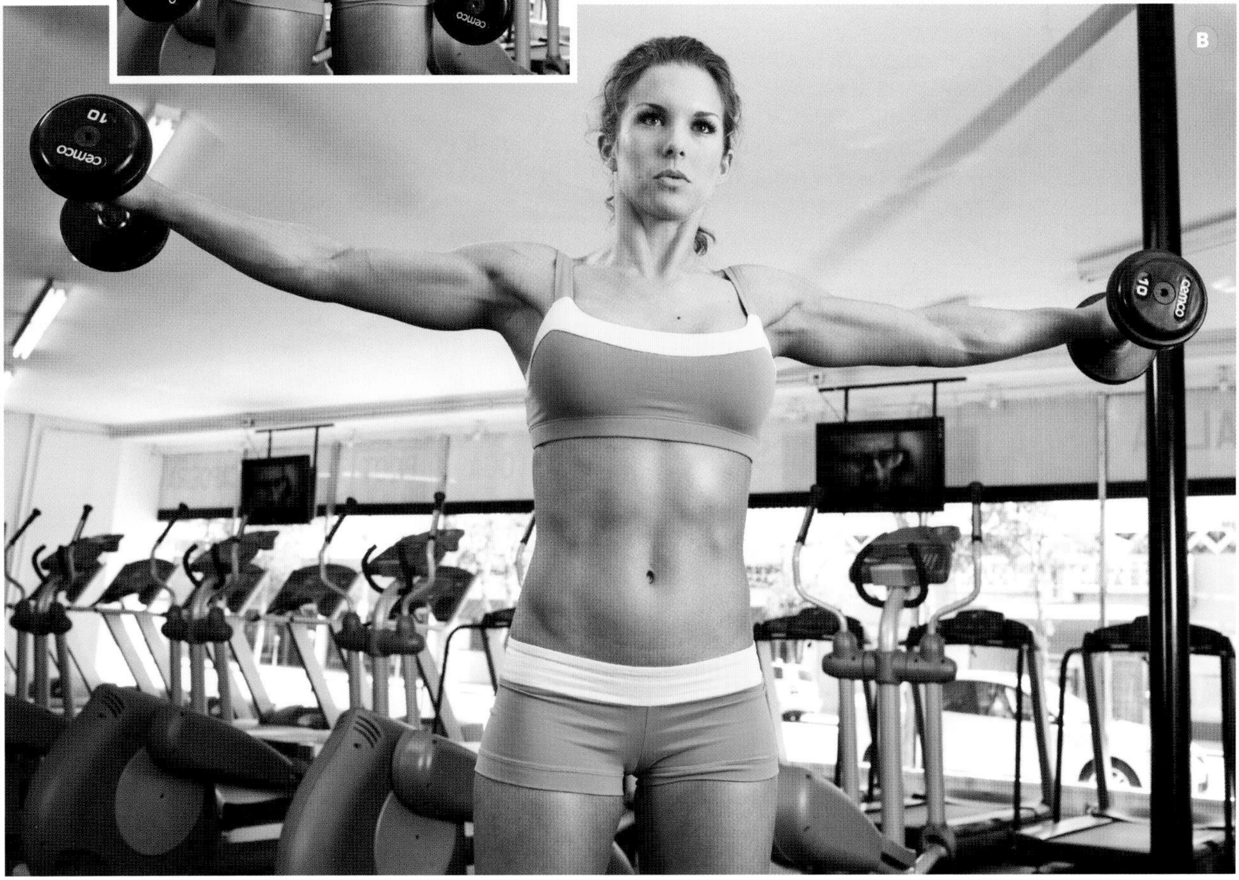

# Standing Dumbbell Overhead Press

INTERMEDIATE/ADVANCED

***Muscles Worked:*** *lateral and anterior deltoid; upper fibers of the trapezius; upper fibers of the pectoralis major; lower fibers of trapezius and rhomboids as stabilizers*

## Technique

1. Standing with feet hip-width apart, legs straight but not locked, hold a dumbbell in each hand just above shoulder height. Elbows are bent and pointing down toward the floor, forearms parallel to each other, wrists straight and palms facing each other.
2. Balance your bodyweight so it's evenly distributed between toes and heels of both feet.
3. Contract abdominal muscles to bring spine to a neutral position, chest lifted and shoulders relaxed.
4. Press shoulder blades together and down, then straighten arms overhead without locking elbows or cocking wrists. Keep weights in your peripheral vision at the top of the lift.
5. Slowly bend elbows and lower to start position.

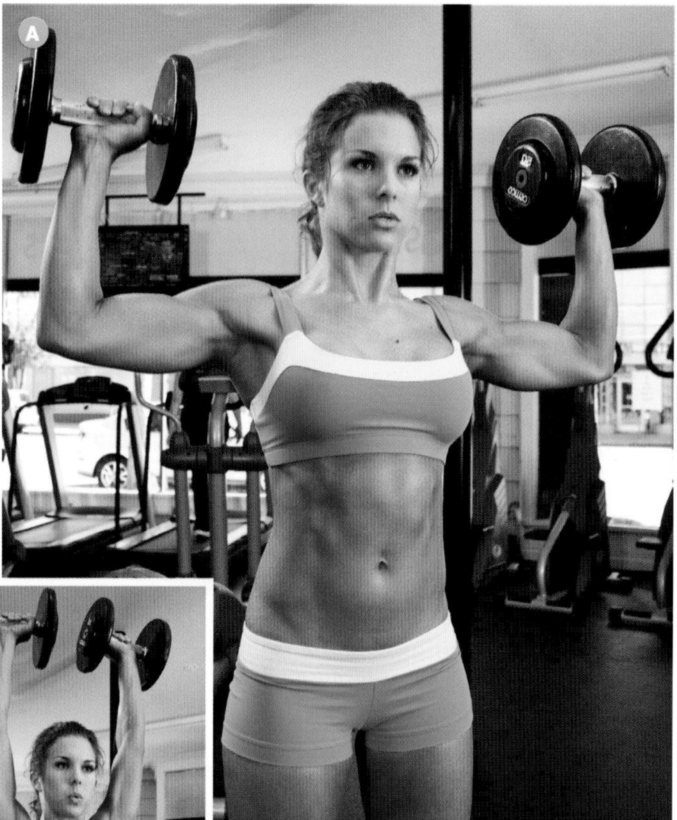


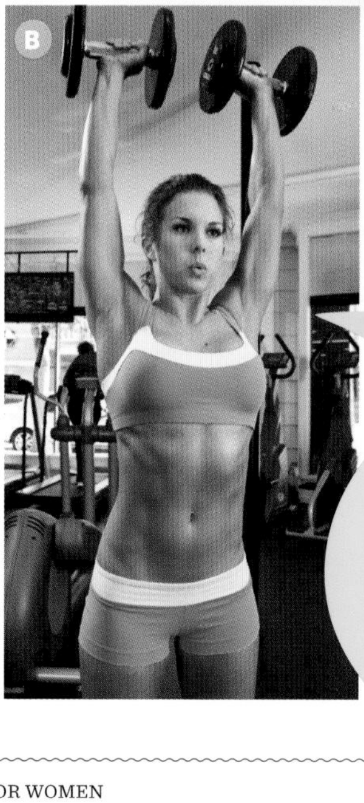


## Trainer's tips

- Your legs should be at least hip-width apart, knees slightly bent.
- As you press dumbbells upward, avoid leaning backward into your heels or rounding your shoulders. These are common errors if the weight is too heavy or if you don't stabilize your position by setting your shoulder blades.
- Don't lock elbows at the top. Straightening your arms more won't increase the benefit.
- For variety, alternate the press-up, raising one arm overhead at a time.

### Inside Edge

***To get the final squeeze on your shoulders, once arms are straight, follow a slightly narrowing path back, aligning arms with shoulder joint.***

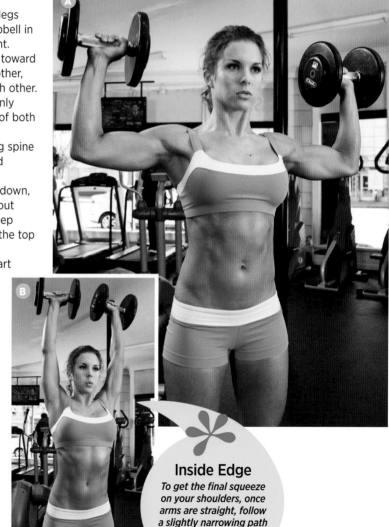

# Dumbbell Upright Row

INTERMEDIATE/ADVANCED

***Muscles Worked:*** *lateral and posterior deltoid; upper trapezius; lower trapezius and rhomboids as stabilizers*

## Technique

1. Holding a dumbbell in each hand with arms hanging on the outside of your thighs and palms facing back, stand with feet hip-width apart, knees slightly bent, quadriceps firm to maintain leg stability, bodyweight balanced equally over both feet.
2. Contract your abdominal muscles, bringing spine to a neutral position, tailbone pointing toward floor, chest lifted and shoulders relaxed.
3. Bend elbows out and up to shoulder height, keeping elbows wide, forearms parallel and wrists neutral so at the top of the lift, your knuckles point down toward the floor.
4. Pause, then straighten arms to start position without rounding shoulders or releasing back muscles.

## Trainer's tips

- Keep elbows wide; using a narrow pulling grip can impinge shoulder muscles. This variation is not only safe, it really hones in on both the shoulder and upper back muscles.
- Keep forearm muscles active and wrists neutral so the weights don't just hang. In the final position, your arms will form an upside-down, modified "goal-post position," with dumbbells aligned with forearms, wrists and shoulders.
- Only lift to shoulder height — any higher may place tension on shoulders and neck.
- For variety, do the same exercise using a barbell and keeping the grip wide, or alternate lifting one dumbbell at a time.

**Inside Edge**

***Keep shoulders down and away from your ears without hunching; press shoulder blades down for the entire exercise.***

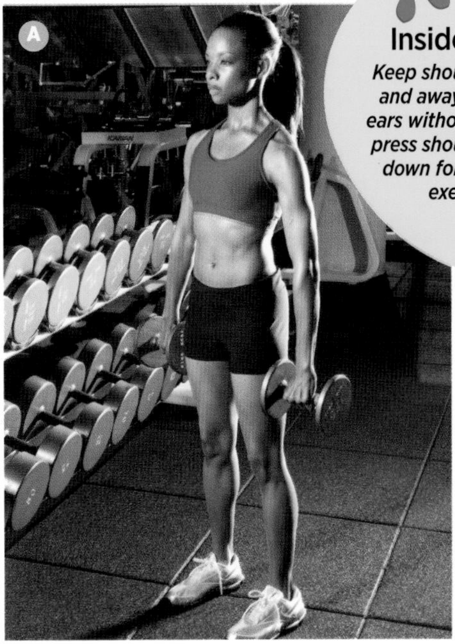


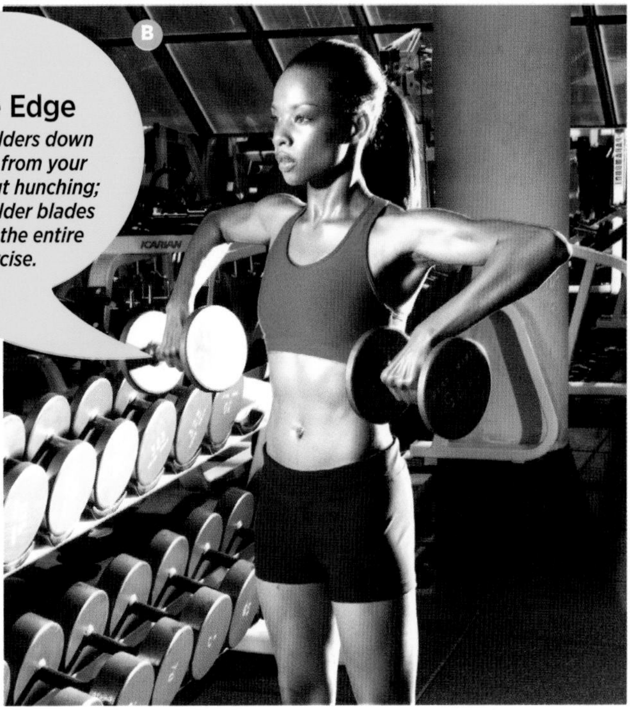

## Beginner Workouts

***Directions:** This is a progressive, six-week program. Do the listed exercises twice a week.*

| WEEK | EXERCISE | SETS | REPS |
|---|---|---|---|
| 1 & 2 | Seated Machine Press | 1–2 | 10–15 |
| | Seated Dumbbell Lateral Raise | 1–2 | 10–12 |
| | Front Raise | 1–2 | 10–15 |
| 3 & 4 | Seated Dumbbell Overhead Press | 1–2 | 10–12 |
| | Seated Lateral Raise | 1–2 | 10–12 |
| | Front Raise | 1–2 | 10–15 |
| 5 & 6 | Seated Dumbbell Overhead or Machine Press | 2 | 10–15 |
| | Front Raise | 2 | 8–12 |
| | Prone Flye | 1–2 | 8–12 |

**Notes**

*Rest 45–60 seconds between sets. At the end of 6 weeks, progress to intermediate workouts if you're ready.*

## Intermediate Workouts

***Directions:** This is a progressive, six-week program using moderate weight. Do the exercises listed twice a week. Adjust the number of reps if you're using lighter or heavier weight.*

| WEEK | EXERCISE | SETS | REPS |
|---|---|---|---|
| 1 & 2 | Standing Dumbbell Overhead Press | 2–3 | 10–15 |
| | Standing Dumbbell Lateral Raise | 2–3 | 10–15 |
| | Front Raise | 2–3 | 10–15 |
| | Prone Flye | 2–3 | 10–15 |
| 3 & 4 | Standing Dumbbell Overhead Press | 2–3 | 10–12 |
| | ***Superset:*** | 2 | |
| | Standing Dumbbell | | |
| | Lateral Raise | | 8–12 |
| | Front Raise | | 8–12 |
| | Bent-Over Standing Rear Flye | 2 | 8–12 |
| 5 & 6 | Dumbbell Upright Row | 2–3 | 8–12 |
| | Incline Side-Lying Raise | 2–3 | 10–12 |
| | Prone Flye | 2–3 | 10–15 |
| | (use incline bench) | | |
| | Front Raise | 2–3 | 8–12 |

**Notes**

*Rest 60–90 seconds between sets. At the end of six weeks, progress to advanced workouts if you're ready.*

## Advanced Workouts

***Directions:*** ***Perform two workouts a week, choosing from the following programs. These programs are based on moderate weight. If you're using light or heavy weight, adjust your reps.***

| EXERCISE | SETS | REPS |
|---|---|---|
| *Workout 1* | | |
| ***Superset:*** | 3 | |
| Barbell Overhead Press | | 10–12 |
| Bent-Over High Row | | 10–12 |
| ***Alternate one rep of each for each set:*** | 3 | |
| Standing Dumbbell Lateral Raise<br>Front Raise | | 10–12 |
| Bent-Over Standing Rear Flye | 3 | 10–12 |
| *Workout 2* | | |
| ***Superset:*** | 3 | |
| Dumbbell Upright Row | | 10–15 |
| Standing Dumbbell Lateral Raise | | 12–15 |
| Bent-Over High Row | 3 | 10–12 |
| ***Superset:*** | 3 | |
| Standing DumbbellOverhead Press | | 10–12 |
| Front Raise | | 10–12 |
| *Workout 3* | | |
| ***Superset:*** | 3 | |
| Bent-Over High Row or<br>Wide-Grip Upright Row | | 8–12 |
| Standing Dumbbell Lateral Raise | | 8–12 |
| Front Raise | | 8–12 |
| Barbell Overhead Press | 3 | 8–12 |
| Bent-Over Standing Rear Flye | 1st* | 12–15 |
| **To pyramid sets, increase weight as you decrease reps* | *2nd* | *10–12* |

***Notes***

*Rest 60–90 seconds between sets.*

## Can't-Get-to-the-Gym Workouts

***Directions:*** ***Do the following exercises when you want to work out at home or on the road. Change the order for variety.***

| EXERCISE | SETS | REPS |
|---|---|---|
| *Workout 1* | | |
| Seated* or Standing Overhead Press | 2–3 | 10–15 |
| Seated Dumbbell Lateral Raise* or | 2–3 | 10–15 |
| Standing Dumbbell Lateral Raise | 2–3 | 10–12 |
| ***Intermediate and Advanced:*** | | |
| Superset with Front Raise | | 10–12 |
| Front Raise* | 2 | 10–15 |
| *Workout 2* | | |
| Seated Dumbbell Overhead Press* | 2 | 10–12 |
| ***or Superset:*** | 3 | |
| Dumbbell Upright Row | | 10–12 |
| Bent-Over High Row with dumbbells | | 10–12 |
| Seated Dumbbell Lateral Raise* or<br>Bent-Over Standing Rear Flye | 2–3 | 10–15<br>10–12 |
| Front Raise* | 2–3 | 10–12 |

***Notes***

*Rest 60–90 seconds between sets. If you're a beginner, do only the exercises marked with an asterisk (*).*